THE ESSENTIAL ALKALINE DIET COOKBOOK

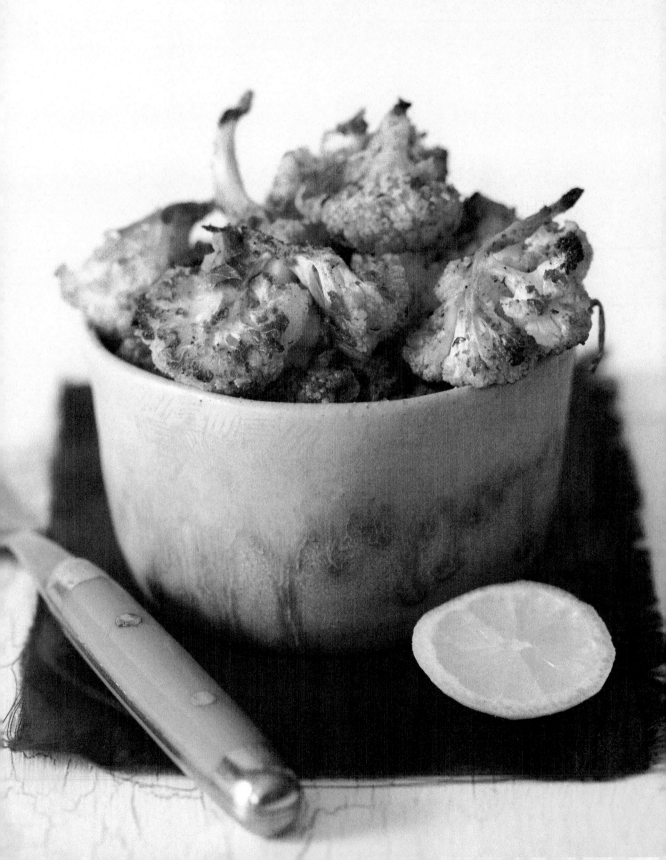

the ESSENTIAL
ALKALINE
DIET COOKBOOK

150 ALKALINE RECIPES
TO BRING YOUR BODY BACK TO BALANCE

ROCKRIDGE
PRESS

ISBN: Print 978-1-62315-523-0 | eBook 978-1-62315-524-7

QUICK START GUIDE

Can't wait to get started?
Follow these five quicksteps, and you'll be on your way to
improved health and delicious eating.

QUICKSTEP ONE

Get out your blender, food processor, and other fun kitchen gadgets.
You're going to use them!

QUICKSTEP TWO

Look in the pantry, the refrigerator, and the freezer to see what you already
have on hand. Make a list, so you'll know what you have and what you need.

QUICKSTEP THREE

Choose a recipe that appeals to you and
also uses ingredients that you have on hand.

QUICKSTEP FOUR

Make a recipe! Try a smoothie, dessert, or quick snack. Let your
taste buds be the judge—you'll see how delicious this food really is.

QUICKSTEP FIVE

Go through the rest of this book and identify five recipes you want
to try first. Be forewarned, it will be tough to choose only five!

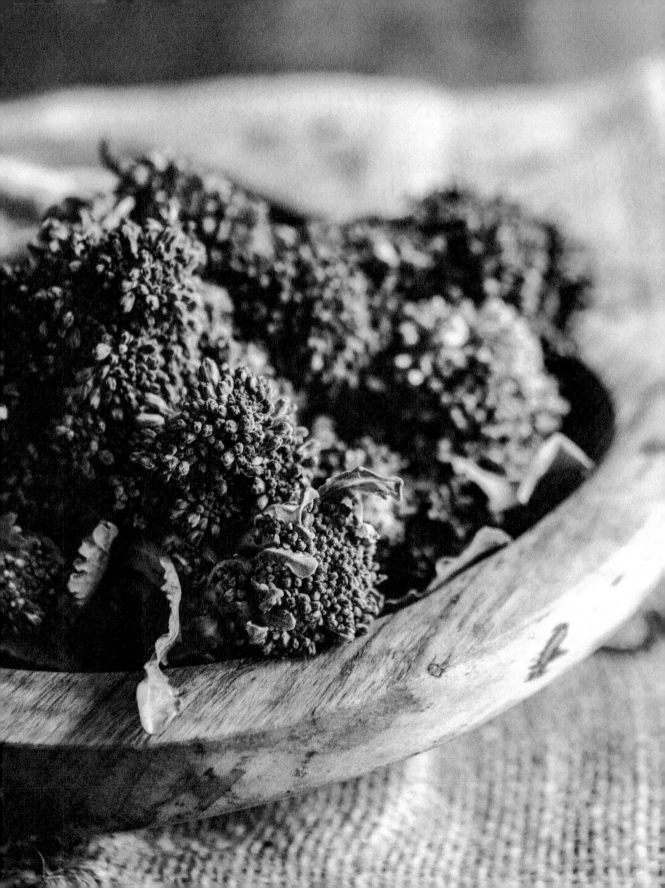

CONTENTS

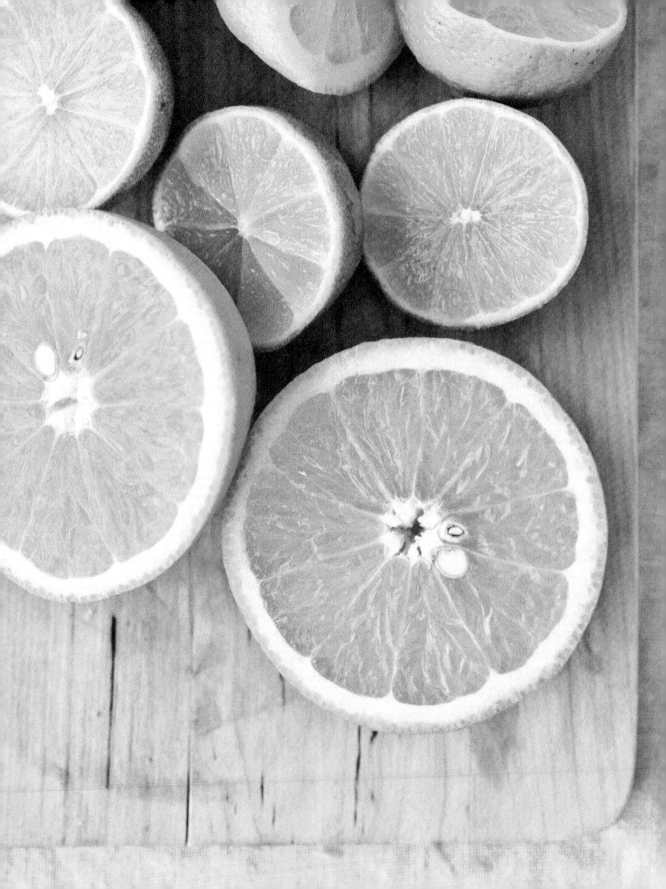

INTRODUCTION

Think of a time when you're woken up in the middle of the night with a bad case of indigestion. It feels like your stomach lining and esophagus are burning. You know the pain is from an overabundance of acid, so you take an antacid. The antacid neutralizes the acid in your stomach by regulating the acid-alkaline balance. The burning pain stops and your body returns to normal.

But what happens if you have an acid imbalance in another part of your body—a part that doesn't give you a painful warning signal? How would you know your body is being damaged? Unlike the burning feeling of indigestion, if your blood or urine is too acidic, you won't necessarily know it. Your body could have too much acid right now, and you'd have no way of knowing until it shows up in the form of a disease or illness.

Although the human body has an amazing ability to regulate the acid-alkaline balance in the blood through our lungs and kidneys, it takes a toll. If those organs are busy fighting an overabundance of acid in order to keep a normal acid-alkaline balance, then they're less likely to be fighting off other problems.

The human body is designed to be slightly alkaline, and at one time it was. Over the course of human evolution, there have been considerable changes in the acid load in our diets. Back in the hunter-gatherer days, there was no Starbucks, or fast-food drive-through. We didn't drink wine or beer, or eat triple-meat pizzas and chili-cheese fries.

Our modern societies have caused the human diet to become imbalanced. The proportion of potassium to sodium is reversed, and we don't get enough magnesium or potassium. We eat too little fiber, and too much saturated fat and refined sugar. Add that to a diet high in animal protein, and it's a recipe for disaster. These foods cause an overabundance of acid in our bodies, which many health professionals suspect can lead to disease.

The Essential Alkaline Diet and Cookbook has two goals:

- To educate and inform you about which foods in your diet are acidic.
- To offer 150 recipes demonstrating how easy and delicious it is to reduce or eliminate acidic foods and switch to an alkaline diet.

The Alkaline Diet has a number of health benefits, including improved bone health, lowered cholesterol and blood pressure, improved cardiovascular health, improved memory and cognition, and better-functioning kidneys. People following this diet tend to lose weight, and feel better. It's a low-sodium, low-sugar, low-fat, high-fiber, antioxidant-rich diet that also happens to be delicious. Plus, you won't be waking up in the middle of the night from acid indigestion!

PART 1
GETTING STARTED

● ● ● ●

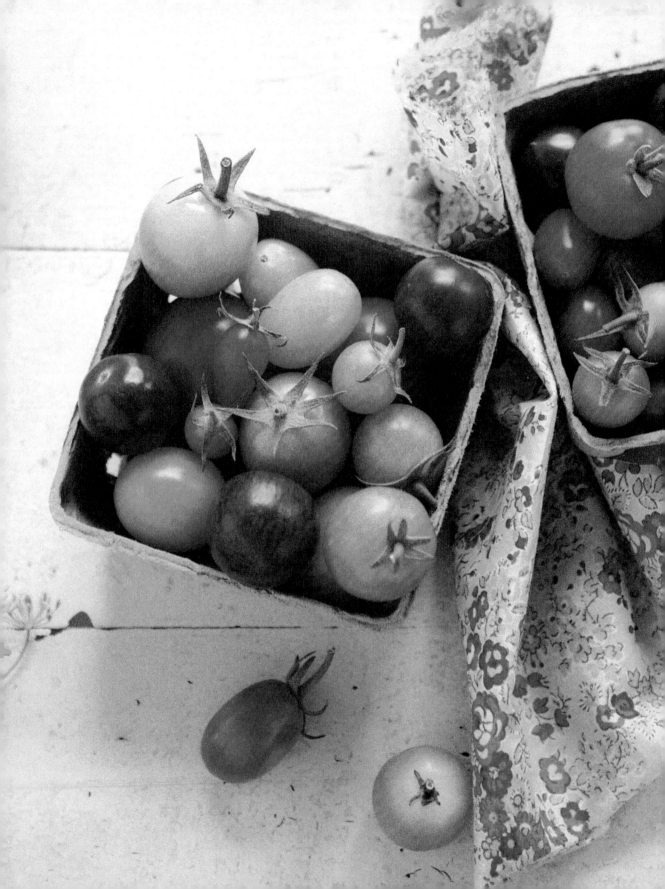

1

ALKALINE DIET BASICS

WHAT IS THE ALKALINE DIET?

The human body is designed to maintain a carefully regulated pH balance by eliminating excess acid. The Standard American Diet focuses mainly on things like white flour, sugar, animal products, and alcohol. Our bodies can handle a certain amount of these foods, but when we overeat acidifying items and don't eat enough of the foods that support our body's ability to neutralize the acid, we become imbalanced. The body is, at times, unable to eliminate excess acid in order to maintain an optimal balance. Some experts believe that it's this imbalance that leads to various illnesses and diseases.

The Alkaline Diet emphasizes foods that promote alkalinity in the blood and urine. These foods include fruits, vegetables, and certain whole grains. This diet balances acidifying foods and alkalizing foods, so that the body functions more effectively.

WHAT IS PH?

In chemistry, the pH scale is used to determine whether water-based mixtures are acidic, basic, or neutral.

••• What Is Alkaline Water?

The term *alkaline water* refers to the pH level of the water. Anything that is alkaline has a pH over 7. So, if the pH of the water is 7.5, you can say it's alkaline water. If it's 6, it's not alkaline water. And, like many terms that have scientific roots, *alkaline water* has been quickly adopted by the advertising crowd. There are many water-alkalizing contraptions available for sale, as well as bottled alkaline water. But, is it necessary?

Most water is actually neutral, with a pH of 7. However, a lot depends on the water's source. Some cities have water that is slightly acidic, and others have slightly alkaline water.

There is no evidence that alkaline water affects the alkalinity of your blood or urine, which is what this diet focuses on.

Researchers Jamie A. Koufman and Nikki Johnston, in the Annals of Otology, Rhinology & Laryngology, have shown that drinking alkaline water with a pH of 8.8 reduces acid reflux. If you suffer from acid reflux, this might be worth a try. The alkaline water may neutralize the acid balance in your stomach to help reduce acid reflux.

As to whether or not you need to drink water that is specifically alkalized, there's no real reason to do so. Regular filtered water is sufficient to hydrate your body and keep your organs healthy.

A substance that is neither acidic nor basic is neutral. The pH scale, ranging from 0 to 14, measures how acidic or basic a substance is. Higher numbers mean a substance is more alkaline (for our purposes, "basic" and "alkaline" mean the same thing) or basic, and lower numbers mean that the substance is more acidic.

A pH of 7 is neutral.

A pH less than 7 is acidic.

A pH greater than 7 is alkaline.

Some foods included in the Alkaline Diet may have an acidic pH (like lemons), but have an alkalizing effect on the body. So, you can't simply determine whether to eat a certain food just by looking at its pH level (more on this later). To help you sort through this, this book includes extensive food charts. By the time you've read *The Essential Alkaline Diet Cookbook*, you'll have a good sense of what foods to eat and which ones to avoid.

HOW FOOD AFFECTS YOUR BODY

The way most people in the Western world eat results in excess acid production after the food is broken down. The result is that the urine can become slightly too acidic, which indicates an overload of acid. Not enough to kill us, but enough to cause an imbalance that can lead to disease.

This happens as a result of foods that are too high in fat, protein, and sugars. When your body metabolizes these foods, acid byproducts form. As you might remember from high school chemistry—or from popping antacids when you feel heartburn—the way to neutralize acid is to combine it with a base. So, to reduce the acid burden, your body uses alkaline minerals to link to the excess acid so the body can eliminate the acid. In a healthy person, the system works to keep the body in a slightly alkaline range (a pH of 7.35 to 7.45). If your diet is very imbalanced, with too much acid and not enough alkalizing minerals, the body can't eliminate the acid byproducts. They build up in the cells of your organs and reduce the efficiency and effectiveness of your body's function.

It's not just the foods we eat. Pollution, viruses, bacteria, and health problems add extra strain on our bodies. To combat the physical stressors, the body releases stress hormones, such as cortisol, adrenaline, and insulin. Your body reacts by slowing digestion. The result is that the food you eat sits longer in your stomach and isn't digested well. So, your body doesn't obtain the optimum amount of nutrients from the food to help it rebuild and repair.

Eating too much acid-producing food wreaks real havoc on your entire body. It has to work harder to maintain a healthy pH balance. Doing so depletes the body's reserves of important minerals and causes the release of stress hormones that affect the body and the mind—not to mention the weight gain and other health problems that come from eating the Standard American Diet.

WHY THE ALKALINE DIET HELPS

For the body to effectively maintain its slightly alkaline balance, it needs a rich supply of alkalizing minerals. And, we need to eat foods that don't overwhelm the body's natural ability to get rid of acid.

The Alkaline Diet works in two ways:

- It eliminates foods that have an acidifying effect on your body.
- It adds nutrients that help repair your body.

In a study published in the *Journal of Environmental and Public Health*, researcher Gerry K. Schwalfenberg found that an alkaline diet resulted in a number of health benefits, some of which include:

1. The increased amounts of fruits and vegetables in an alkaline diet improve the body's potassium-sodium ratio. This may benefit bone health and muscle tone, and lessen other chronic illnesses, like hypertension and stroke.

2. An alkaline diet can help slow the natural loss of muscle mass that comes with aging.

3. Many alkaline foods are rich in magnesium, a mineral that activates vitamin D, which benefits our bones, kidneys, and hearts, among other things.

If you're recovering from an illness or chronic condition, the Alkaline Diet will infuse your body with much-needed nutrition to start the healing process, and it removes the additional stressors that a bad diet can create.

For instance, according to the National Institutes of Health, diet is one of several factors that can contribute to kidney stone formation. Kidney stones can form when substances in the urine—such as calcium and phosphorus—become highly concentrated. After the body uses what it needs from the food we eat for rebuilding, the waste products in the bloodstream are carried to the kidneys and excreted as urine.

It makes sense, then, that if our diet minimizes these harmful substances and the kidneys don't have to work as hard to balance the acid-alkaline level in your body, they'll be able to avoid kidney stones. Also, if your thyroid isn't busy handling stress hormones released because of the food you eat, it will be better able to function. Our thyroids regulate many of the hormones in the body, including those that affect our metabolism. In this way, you can achieve and sustain a healthy immune system and overall health.

••• The 80/20 Rule

Eighty percent of your food should come from the "Go" list of alkalizing foods (see page 23). However, throughout *The Essential Alkaline Diet Cookbook*, you'll find information that indicates when certain foods should be "part of your 20 percent." This means it's okay to include some mildly acidic foods in your diet, but they shouldn't be more than 20 percent of your overall diet. Those recipes alert you, so it will be easy to stay on track.

HOW TO FOLLOW THE ALKALINE DIET

By now you may be convinced that the Alkaline Diet is the way to go. But what does it actually *look* like every day? What will you actually eat?

Remember that the goal of the Alkaline Diet is twofold:

1. To eliminate or reduce foods that cause a buildup of acid in the body.

2. To add foods high in important minerals that help your body alkalize itself.

Following are some tips for success:

- Eat at least two cups of alkaline greens (kale, mustard or turnip greens, collards, or endive) daily. Lettuce is fine, but not in place of alkaline greens. Grated daikon radish is a wonderful alkalinizing condiment.

- Add miso and seaweed to soups and other dishes as both a digestive aid and an alkalizer. You can also find seaweed snacks in most grocery stores and markets these days. These crunchy treats are delicious and they add beneficial alkalizing minerals to your diet.

- Eat more alkalizing grains like oats, quinoa, and wild rice.

- Enjoy liberal amounts of fresh fruits, especially watermelon.

ACIDIC FOODS THAT ARE ALKALIZING

As you read through the recipes, you'll find some foods on the "Go" list that are very acidic (like lemons and apple cider vinegar). You might be wondering how some foods can be acidic outside the body but have alkalizing effects when eaten. The answer lies in the "ash" content of the food when burned. When a food is burned—this is something done by food scientists in a controlled environment; your barbecue isn't likely to yield trustworthy results, no matter how badly burned your burgers get—if the resulting ash residue is more alkaline than acid, it's considered an alkalizing food. The reason is that when our body digests food, it undergoes oxidation, which is similar to burning, and the result is what determines whether the end product is alkaline or acid.

ACID-FORMING FOODS TO AVOID

On the Alkaline Diet you'll want to avoid any animal products (meat, dairy, fish, and eggs). Also avoid alcohol, coffee, and black tea, as they are highly acidic. Similarly, refined sugars of any kind should be avoided. And, as most grains have an acidifying effect on the body, they should be avoided, too.

Following is a more extensive list of "No Go" acid-forming foods to avoid.

Acidifying Beans, Legumes, and Milks

- Rice milk
- Soy milk
- Soy beans
- Unsprouted beans

Acidifying Fats and Oils

- Avocado oil
- Flax oil
- Olive oil
- Butter
- Hemp oil
- Safflower oil
- Canola oil
- Lard
- Sunflower oil
- Corn oil

Acidifying Fruits

- Blueberries
- Cranberries
- Canned or glazed fruits
- Currants

Acidifying Grains and Grain Products

- Amaranth
- Bran, wheat
- Cornstarch
- Barley
- Bread
- Crackers, soda
- Bran, oat
- Corn
- Flour, wheat

- Flour, white
- Hemp seed flour
- Kamut
- Noodles
- Oatmeal
- Oats, rolled
- Pasta
- Rice cakes
- Rice, white
- Rye
- Spelt
- Wheat
- Wheat germ

Acidifying Nuts and Butters

- Cashews
- Legumes
- Peanut butter
- Peanuts
- Pecans
- Tahini
- Walnuts

Acidifying Sweeteners

- Carob
- Corn syrup
- Sugar

Acidifying Vegetables

- Corn
- Lentils
- Olives

All Alcohol

- Beer
- Hard liquor
- Spirits
- Wine

All Animal Protein

- Beef
- Eggs
- Fish
- Lamb
- Organ meats
- Pork
- Poultry
- Rabbit
- Sausage
- Shellfish
- Venison

Dairy

- Butter
- Cheese, processed
- Ice cream
- Yogurt

Other Foods

- Black tea
- Cocoa
- Coffee
- Ketchup
- Mustard
- Pepper
- Soft drinks
- Vinegar

••• Curbing Cravings

After reading the "No Go" list of foods to avoid, you're probably wondering how on earth you're going to avoid eating (or craving!) all those foods. Not to worry; following is a list of tips for curbing cravings.

- **Plan ahead.** If you know you are going somewhere where there will be lots of tempting foods, bring your own. Or, make something delicious from this book and promise yourself you can have it when you get home. It's much easier to pass up an unhealthy item if you know you have something delicious waiting for you later.

- **Plan your 20 percent.** If there is a food on the "No Go" list that you can't live without, plan to include it as part of your 20 percent.

- **Swap it out.** Many of the recipes in this book are healthier versions of unhealthy favorites. Don't think you're giving up your favorite foods. You're really just eating healthier versions.

- **Picture your payoff.** Get a photograph or some other visual reminder of why you're making these healthy changes in the first place. A photo of your baby granddaughter placed on the refrigerator can remind you why you want to live a long, healthy life.

- **Watch out for food ads!** Restaurants and food manufacturers spend millions of advertising dollars trying to get you to eat their food. So, if you're on the couch watching TV and suddenly craving food, be aware you're being manipulated. Get mad! Say to yourself, "I know you want me to eat your food, but I value my healthy choices more." Then, go get a healthy snack.

- **Reward yourself.** Keep track of how many times you successfully fight a craving. After a set number of times, give yourself a non-food reward, like a night out at the movies or a new book you've been wanting to read.

ALKALINE FOODS TO ENJOY

As a general rule, you'll want to focus on eating fruits and vegetables (with the exception of a few items.) There are a few grains, like quinoa, on the "Go" list. As far as oil goes, you'll notice recipes call for coconut oil and sesame oil. You can get both at your regular grocery store. Also, the baking recipes often call for coconut flour, which is also available at regular markets these days or can easily be procured online. Check the Resources section for more sources for these foods. Following is the list of "Go" foods to enjoy!

Alkalizing Fruits

- Apple
- Apricot
- Avocado
- Banana
- Berries
- Blackberries
- Cantaloupe
- Cherry, sour
- Coconut, fresh
- Currant
- Date, dried
- Fig, dried
- Grape
- Grapefruit
- Honeydew melon
- Lemon
- Lime
- Muskmelon
- Nectarine
- Orange
- Peach
- Pear
- Pineapple
- Raisins
- Raspberry
- Rhubarb
- Strawberry
- Tangerine
- Tomato
- Tropical fruits
- Umeboshi plum
- Watermelon

Alkalizing Proteins

- Almond
- Chestnut
- Millet
- Tempeh, fermented
- Tofu, fermented
- Whey protein powder

Alkalizing Seasonings and Spices

- Chili pepper
- Cinnamon
- Curry
- Ginger
- Herbs, all
- Miso
- Mustard
- Sea salt
- Tamari

Alkalizing Sweeteners

- Stevia

Alkalizing Vegetables

- Alfalfa
- Barley grass
- Beet greens
- Beets
- Broccoli
- Cabbage
- Carrot
- Cauliflower
- Celery
- Chard greens
- Chlorella
- Collard greens
- Cucumber
- Daikon
- Dandelion
- Dandelion root
- Dulce
- Edible flowers
- Eggplant
- Fermented vegetables
- Garlic
- Green beans
- Green peas
- Kale
- Kohlrabi
- Kombu
- Lettuce
- Maitake
- Mushroom
- Mustard greens
- Nori
- Onions
- Parsnip
- Pea
- Pepper
- Pumpkin
- Radish
- Reishi
- Rutabaga
- Sea vegetables
- Shiitake
- Spinach, green
- Spirulina
- Sprouts
- Sweet potato
- Tomato
- Wakame
- Watercress
- Wheat grass
- Wild greens

Other

- Apple cider vinegar
- Bee pollen
- Fresh fruit juice
- Green juices
- Lecithin granules
- Molasses, blackstrap
- Probiotic cultures
- Soured dairy products
- Vegetable juices
- Water, alkaline antioxidant
- Water, mineral

••• Surprise, It's Acidic!

As you have seen, most fruits and vegetables are on the "Go" list because of their alkalizing effect on your body, but there are some foods on the "No Go" list that you might be surprised to see there. Remember, it's not whether a food has an acidic pH, but rather its effect on the body. Following is a surprising list of foods that are acidifying and should be avoided.

- Barley
- Black olives
- Blueberries
- Bulgur
- Chocolate
- Corn
- Cranberry
- Hazelnut

- Oats
- Peanut butter
- Peanuts
- Pecans
- Pistachios
- Pomegranates
- Soybean

- Soy milk
- Tofu
- Walnut
- Wheat
- White pasta
- White rice
- Whole wheat

Also, use the following foods sparingly:

- Black beans
- Brown rice

- Chickpeas
- Pinto beans

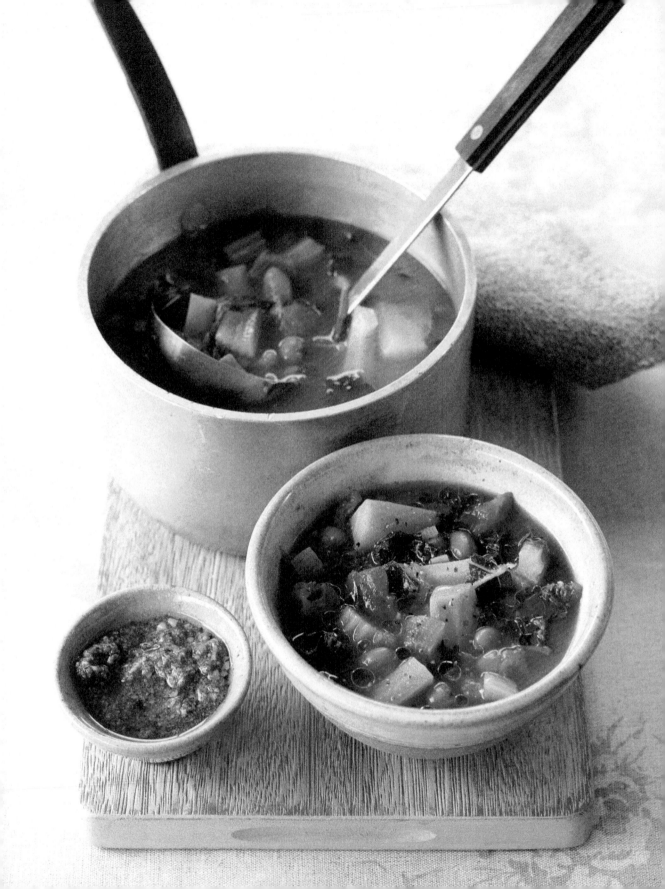

THIRTY–DAY MEAL PLANS

HOW TO USE THE MEAL PLANS

To make it easy for you to follow the Alkaline Diet targeted to specific health issues, we've created three 30-day meal plans to guide you.

PLAN 1 The Immunity-Boost Plan
which is helpful if you are battling cancer or an autoimmune disease.

PLAN 2 The Thyroid-Support Plan
to help balance an over- or underactive thyroid.

PLAN 3 The Kidney-Support Plan
for those struggling with kidney stones or other related issues.

The Alkaline Diet will help ease the strain your body faces as it fights these specific conditions.

To make it even easier, all recipes included in the meal plans are found in this book. These are only guidelines so feel free to swap out recipes, as desired. General suggestions for how to create your own specialized diet are found at the beginning of each meal plan. Just remember to follow the 80/20 rule!

THE IMMUNITY–BOOST PLAN

This diet plan is designed to boost your immune system. Even if you're not facing cancer or an autoimmune condition, it's still a great way to help prevent a cold or the flu. The key to an immune-boost diet is to choose a wide variety of different-colored foods. That's why it's also called "eating the rainbow." The reason for this strategy is that colored foods contain micronutrients. These are vitamins and minerals the body needs to stay healthy. So, for the next 30 days, taste the rainbow.

DAY ONE

Breakfast: Good Morning Popeye
Lunch: South-of-the-Border Salad
Dinner: You Won't Miss the Clams Chowder
Snack: Banana Candy Coins

DAY TWO

Breakfast: Basic Green Smoothie
Lunch: Salad on a Stick
Dinner: The Mexican Bowl
Snack: Warm Peach Cobbler

DAY THREE

Breakfast: Garden Pancakes
Lunch: Better Than Chicken Soup
Dinner: Championship Chili
Snack: Crispy Rice Treats

DAY FOUR

Breakfast: Banana Nut Bread Smoothie
Lunch: Eggplant Rollups
Dinner: The Asian Bowl
Snack: Herbed Crackers and Healthy Hummus

DAY FIVE

Breakfast: Banana Muffins
Lunch: Spicy Sesame Noodle Salad
Dinner: Curried Eggplant
Snack: No-Bake Fig Newtons

DAY SIX

Breakfast: Tropical Piña Colada Smoothie
Lunch: Sushi Hand Roll
Dinner: Grilled Vegetable Stack
Snack: Oven-Baked Onion Rings

DAY SEVEN

Breakfast: The "Can This Be Kale?" Smoothie
Lunch: The Indian Bowl
Dinner: Vegetable Potpie
Snack: Szechuan Green Beans

DAY EIGHT

Breakfast: Summer Fruit Salad with Lime and Mint
Lunch: Warm Ginger, Garlic, Lemon Smoothie
Dinner: Cinco de Mayo Casserole
Snack: Baked Sweet Potato and Apple

Breakfast: Spaghetti Squash Hash Browns
Lunch: Warm Spinach Salad
Dinner: Angel Hair Pasta with Hearty Tomato Sauce
Snack: Date-Spice Pudding

Breakfast: Liquid Guacamole
Lunch: Pad Thai Salad
Dinner: The Lady and the Tramp Bowl
Snack: Vegetable Chips

Breakfast: Almond-Quinoa Muffins
Lunch: Spicy Orange-Broccoli Salad
Dinner: Stuffed Peppers
Snack: Sweet Potato Fries

Breakfast: Breakfast Fajitas
Lunch: Mango-Barbecue Sliders
Dinner: Emerald Forest Salad
Snack: Self-Frosting Carrot Cake

Breakfast: Banana Muffins
Lunch: Salad in Your Hand
Dinner: The Hawaiian Bowl
Snack: Pumpkin-Rhubarb Pie

Breakfast: Brown Rice Porridge
Lunch: Sushi Hand Roll
Dinner: The Fight It Off Bowl
Snack: Better Than Girl Scout Cookies

Breakfast: Winter Fruit Compote with Figs and Ginger
Lunch: The Rose Bowl
Dinner: Date Night Garlic Bake
Snack: Movie Night Cauliflower Popcorn

Breakfast: Better-Than-a-Coffeehouse Pumpkin Drink
Lunch: Asian Cabbage Slaw
Dinner: Layered Ratatouille
Snack: Coconut Ice Cream Sundae

Breakfast: Orange, Peach, Kale Smoothie
Lunch: Avocado-Caprese Salad
Dinner: The Southern Bowl
Snack: Baked Apples and Raisins

Breakfast: Baby Potato Home Fries
Lunch: Thanksgiving Anytime Roasted Vegetables
Dinner: No BS Brussels Sprouts
Snack: Thanksgiving Pudding

Breakfast: Hearty Breakfast Sausage
Lunch: Organic Baby Tomato and Kale Salad
Dinner: Stir-Fry Vegetables
Snack: Don't Slip Banana Splits

DAY TWENTY

Breakfast: Sweet Potato Waffles with Applesauce
Lunch: Avocado, Strawberry, Spinach Salad
Dinner: The Super Bowl
Snack: Snickerdoodle Cookies

DAY TWENTY-ONE

Breakfast: Breakfast Parfait
Lunch: Tea Party Cucumber Sandwiches
Dinner: Summer Dinner Salad
Snack: Summer Afternoon Ice Pops

DAY TWENTY-TWO

Breakfast: Orange You Glad It's Healthy Smoothie
Lunch: Russian Ruby Salad
Dinner: Layered Ratatouille
Snack: The Breakup Bowl

DAY TWENTY-THREE

Breakfast: Pumpkin-Spice Quinoa Casserole
Lunch: Roasted Garlic Cabbage
Dinner: South-of-the-Border Salad
Snack: The Monster Mash

DAY TWENTY-FOUR

Breakfast: Chile-Lime Mango Slaw
Lunch: Under-the-Sea Salad
Dinner: BBB Soup
Snack: Sweet Potato Fries

DAY TWENTY-FIVE

Breakfast: All-American Apple Pie
Lunch: Gazpacho Smoothie
Dinner: Lovers' Lasagna
Snack: Santa's Ginger Snaps

DAY TWENTY-SIX

Breakfast: Grandma's Baked Grapefruit
Lunch: Marinated Vegetables
Dinner: Cinco de Mayo Casserole
Snack: Buffalo Flowers

DAY TWENTY-SEVEN

Breakfast: Brown Rice Porridge
Lunch: Cucumber Soup in a Cup
Dinner: You Won't Miss the Clams Chowder
Snack: The Hollywood Bowl

DAY TWENTY-EIGHT

Breakfast: Baked Apples and Raisins
Lunch: The Mexican Bowl
Dinner: Date Night Garlic Bake
Snack: Sparkling Lime–Asian Pear Green Smoothie

DAY TWENTY-NINE

Breakfast: Tropical Granola
Lunch: Hang Up the Phone Mini-Pizzas
Dinner: The Indian Bowl
Snack: Spinach-Artichoke Dip

DAY THIRTY

Breakfast: Garden Pancakes
Lunch: Roasted Vegetable Salad
Dinner: Layered Ratatouille
Snack: Better Than Girl Scout Cookies

● PLAN 2
THE THYROID–SUPPORT PLAN

To develop a diet that supports your thyroid, follow these guidelines. Avoid gluten! This should be easy, as the foods included on the Alkaline Diet are naturally gluten-free. Also, avoid foods that can be inflammatory, including nightshades (tomatoes, peppers, eggplants). For extra benefit, eat a food every day containing coconut oil, as that tends to support the thyroid. The majority of recipes suggested for this plan contain coconut oil. If a day's plan does not include it, eat a tablespoon of coconut oil by itself to maintain the benefits.

DAY ONE

Breakfast: Tropical Piña Colada Smoothie
Lunch: Sushi Hand Roll
Dinner: The Asian Bowl
Snack: Oven-Baked Onion Rings

DAY TWO

Breakfast: More-Than-a-Mojito Smoothie
Lunch: Szechuan Green Beans
Dinner: Better Than Chicken Soup
Snack: Self-Frosting Carrot Cake

DAY THREE

Breakfast: Orange, Peach, Kale Smoothie
Lunch: Warm Spinach Salad
Dinner: Better Than Chicken Soup
Snack: Santa's Ginger Snaps

DAY FOUR

Breakfast: Basic Green Smoothie
Lunch: Spicy Sesame Noodle Salad
Dinner: You Won't Miss the Clams Chowder
Snack: Oven-Baked Onion Rings

DAY FIVE

Breakfast: Banana Nut Bread Smoothie
Lunch: Spicy Orange-Broccoli Salad
Dinner: Vegetable Potpie
Snack: Banana Candy Coins

DAY SIX

Breakfast: Summer Fruit Salad with Lime and Mint
Lunch: Asian Cabbage Slaw
Dinner: Date Night Garlic Bake
Snack: Buffalo Flowers

DAY SEVEN

Breakfast: Cherry-Chocolate Smoothie
Lunch: Roasted Vegetable Salad
Dinner: No BS Brussels Sprouts
Snack: Chile-Lime Mango Slaw

DAY EIGHT

Breakfast: Good Morning Popeye
Lunch: Sushi Hand Roll
Dinner: Avocado, Strawberry, Spinach Salad
Snack: Mushroom Pâté

DAY NINE

Breakfast: Garden Pancakes
Lunch: Sushi Hand Roll
Dinner: Summer Dinner Salad
Snack: Party Mix

DAY TEN

Breakfast: All-American Apple Pie
Lunch: Spinach-Artichoke Dip
Dinner: Asian Cabbage Slaw
Snack: Mushroom Pâté

DAY ELEVEN

Breakfast: Baby Potato Home Fries
Lunch: Pad Thai Salad
Dinner: The Lazy Bowl
Snack: Valentine's Day Dates

DAY TWELVE

Breakfast: Spaghetti Squash
Hash Browns
Lunch: The Fight It Off Bowl
Dinner: The Lazy Bowl
Snack: Melon Madness

DAY THIRTEEN

Breakfast: Hearty Breakfast Sausage
Lunch: Warm Spinach Salad
Dinner: Spicy Sesame Noodle Salad
Snack: Crispy Rice Treats

DAY FOURTEEN

Breakfast: Brown Rice Porridge
Lunch: Pad Thai Salad
Dinner: The Hawaiian Bowl, made
with Asian Citrus Dressing
Snack: Herbed Crackers

DAY FIFTEEN

Breakfast: Grandma's Baked Grapefruit
Lunch: Quinoa and Avocado Salad
Dinner: The Rose Bowl
Snack: Summer Afternoon Ice Pops

DAY SIXTEEN

Breakfast: Summer Fruit Salad with
Lime and Mint
Lunch: Emerald Forest Salad
Dinner: The Harvest Bowl
Snack: Movie Night Cauliflower
Popcorn

DAY SEVENTEEN

Breakfast: Pumpkin-Spice Quinoa
Casserole
Lunch: BBB Soup
Dinner: No BS Brussels Sprouts
Snack: No-Bake Fig Newtons

DAY EIGHTEEN

Breakfast: The Hollywood Bowl
Lunch: Better Than Chicken Soup
Dinner: Date Night Garlic Bake
Snack: Warm Peach Cobbler

DAY NINETEEN

Breakfast: Orange You Glad It's
Healthy Smoothie
Lunch: Sushi Hand Roll
Dinner: You Won't Miss the
Clams Chowder
Snack: Snickerdoodle Cookies

DAY TWENTY

Breakfast: Winter Fruit Compote with Figs and Ginger
Lunch: Tea Party Cucumber Sandwiches
Dinner: Better Than Chicken Soup
Snack: Better Than Girl Scout Cookies

DAY TWENTY-ONE

Breakfast: Good Morning Popeye
Lunch: Quinoa and Avocado Salad
Dinner: The Comfort Bowl
Snack: Self-Frosting Carrot Cake

DAY TWENTY-TWO

Breakfast: Baby Potato Home Fries
Lunch: Spicy Orange-Broccoli Salad
Dinner: Salad on a Stick
Snack: Baked Apples and Raisins

DAY TWENTY-THREE

Breakfast: All-American Apple Pie
Lunch: Asian Cabbage Slaw
Dinner: Marinated Vegetables
Snack: Cherry-Chocolate Smoothie

DAY TWENTY-FOUR

Breakfast: Cucumber Soup in a Cup
Lunch: Avocado, Strawberry, Spinach Salad
Dinner: Salad on a Stick
Snack: Party Mix

DAY TWENTY-FIVE

Breakfast: Almond-Quinoa Muffins
Lunch: Roasted Vegetable Salad
Dinner: The Hawaiian Bowl, made with Asian Citrus Dressing
Snack: Chile-Lime Mango Slaw

DAY TWENTY-SIX

Breakfast: Banana Muffins
Lunch: Salad in Your Hand
Dinner: Vegetable Potpie
Snack: Don't Slip Banana Splits

DAY TWENTY-SEVEN

Breakfast: Spaghetti Squash Hash Browns
Lunch: Emerald Forest Salad
Dinner: No BS Brussels Sprouts
Snack: Melon Madness

DAY TWENTY-EIGHT

Breakfast: Breakfast Parfait
Lunch: Spicy Sesame Noodle Salad
Dinner: The Super Bowl
Snack: Summer Fruit Crisp

DAY TWENTY-NINE

Breakfast: Brown Rice Porridge
Lunch: Avocado, Strawberry, Spinach Salad
Dinner: Better Than Chicken Soup
Snack: No-Bake Fig Newtons

DAY THIRTY

Breakfast: Baked Sweet Potato and Apple
Lunch: Avocado, Strawberry, Spinach Salad
Dinner: The Lazy Bowl
Snack: Thanksgiving Pudding

● PLAN 3
THE KIDNEY–SUPPORT PLAN

According to Dr. Andrew Weil, "The two most important things you can do to protect your kidney function from further decline are to follow a low-protein diet (no more than 10 to 15 percent of calories from protein), and never allow yourself to become dehydrated." He recommends drinking six to eight glasses of fluids daily—water or mostly water in the form of hot or iced caffeine-free teas or mineral water (flavored or unflavored, but not sweetened).

DAY ONE

Breakfast: Cherry-Chocolate Smoothie
Lunch: The Mexican Bowl
Dinner: Better Than Chicken Soup
Snack: Better Than Girl Scout Cookies

DAY TWO

Breakfast: Good Morning Popeye
Lunch: The Asian Bowl
Dinner: Championship Chili
Snack: Don't Slip Banana Splits

DAY THREE

Breakfast: Banana Nut Bread Smoothie
Lunch: Marinated Vegetables
Dinner: Date Night Garlic Bake
Snack: Coconut Ice Cream Sundae

DAY FOUR

Breakfast: Breakfast Fajitas
Lunch: The Italian Bowl
Dinner: BBB Soup
Snack: Vegetable Chips

DAY FIVE

Breakfast: Garden Pancakes
Lunch: Salad on a Stick
Dinner: The Lady and the Tramp Bowl
Snack: Szechuan Green Beans

DAY SIX

Breakfast: Orange You Glad It's Healthy Smoothie
Lunch: The Super Bowl
Dinner: Curried Eggplant
Snack: Cherry-Chocolate Smoothie

DAY SEVEN

Breakfast: Summer Fruit Salad with Lime and Mint
Lunch: Sushi Hand Roll
Dinner: Stir-Fry Vegetables
Snack: Oven-Baked Onion Rings

DAY EIGHT

Breakfast: Tropical Piña Colada Smoothie
Lunch: Hang Up the Phone Mini-Pizzas
Dinner: The Comfort Bowl
Snack: Chile-Lime Mango Slaw

DAY NINE

Breakfast: Good Morning Popeye
Lunch: Salad in Your Hand
Dinner: Angel Hair Pasta with Hearty Tomato Sauce
Snack: The Breakup Bowl

DAY TEN

Breakfast: Better-Than-a-Coffeehouse Pumpkin Drink
Lunch: Tea Party Cucumber Sandwiches
Dinner: The Mexican Bowl
Snack: Baked Apples and Raisins

DAY ELEVEN

Breakfast: Garden Pancakes
Lunch: Salad on a Stick
Dinner: The Asian Bowl
Snack: Self-Frosting Carrot Cake

DAY TWELVE

Breakfast: Basic Green Smoothie
Lunch: South-of-the-Border Salad
Dinner: Lovers' Lasagna
Snack: Summer Afternoon Ice Pops

DAY THIRTEEN

Breakfast: Tropical Granola
Lunch: Eggplant Rollups
Dinner: Stir-Fry Vegetables
Snack: Buffalo Flowers

DAY FOURTEEN

Breakfast: More-Than-a-Mojito Smoothie
Lunch: Roasted Vegetable Salad
Dinner: Thanksgiving Anytime Roasted Vegetables
Snack: Date-Spice Pudding

DAY FIFTEEN

Breakfast: Summer Fruit Salad with Lime and Mint
Lunch: Tea Party Cucumber Sandwiches
Dinner: The Indian Bowl
Snack: Warm Peach Cobbler

DAY SIXTEEN

Breakfast: Liquid Guacamole
Lunch: Pad Thai Salad
Dinner: Southern Bowl
Snack: Herbed Crackers

DAY SEVENTEEN

Breakfast: Winter Fruit Compote with Figs and Ginger
Lunch: Quinoa and Avocado Salad
Dinner: Vegetable Potpie
Snack: Summer Fruit Crisp

DAY EIGHTEEN

Breakfast: The "Can This Be Kale?" Smoothie
Lunch: Hang Up the Phone Mini-Pizzas
Dinner: The Lazy Bowl
Snack: Banana Candy Coins

DAY NINETEEN

Breakfast: All-American Apple Pie
Lunch: Avocado-Caprese Salad
Dinner: Angel Hair Pasta with Hearty Tomato Sauce
Snack: Coconut Ice Cream Sundae

DAY TWENTY

Breakfast: Orange, Peach, Kale Smoothie
Lunch: Sushi Hand Roll
Dinner: Championship Chili
Snack: Vegetable Chips

DAY TWENTY-ONE

Breakfast: Baby Potato Home Fries
Lunch: Spicy Sesame Noodle Salad
Dinner: Grilled Vegetable Stack
Snack: Baked Apples and Raisins

DAY TWENTY-TWO

Breakfast: Cucumber Soup in a Cup
Lunch: Spicy Orange-Broccoli Salad
Dinner: BBB Soup
Snack: Party Mix

DAY TWENTY-THREE

Breakfast: Breakfast Fajitas
Lunch: Salad in Your Hand
Dinner: Curried Eggplant
Snack: Mushroom Pâté

DAY TWENTY-FOUR

Breakfast: Gazpacho Smoothie
Lunch: Emerald Forest Salad
Dinner: Date Night Garlic Bake
Snack: Sweet Potato Fries

DAY TWENTY-FIVE

Breakfast: Grandma's Baked
Grapefruit
Lunch: Avocado, Strawberry,
Spinach Salad
Dinner: Lovers' Lasagna
Snack: Movie Night Cauliflower
Popcorn

DAY TWENTY-SIX

Breakfast: Sparkling Lime–Asian Pear
Green Smoothie
Lunch: Marinated Vegetables
Dinner: The Indian Bowl
Snack: Melon Madness

DAY TWENTY-SEVEN

Breakfast: Hearty Breakfast Sausage
Lunch: Mango-Barbecue Sliders
Dinner: Better Than Chicken Soup
Snack: The Hollywood Bowl

DAY TWENTY-EIGHT

Breakfast: Warm Ginger, Garlic,
Lemon Smoothie
Lunch: Spinach-Artichoke Dip
Dinner: Summer Dinner Salad
Snack: Roasted Garlic Cabbage

DAY TWENTY-NINE

Breakfast: Mango, Papaya,
Raspberry Smoothie
Lunch: Russian Ruby Salad
Dinner: Stuffed Peppers
Snack: The Breakup Bowl

DAY THIRTY

Breakfast: Sweet Potato Waffles with
Apple Sauce
Lunch: Asian Cabbage Slaw
Dinner: Championship Chili
Snack: Coconut Ice Cream Sundae

PART 2
THE RECIPES

● ● ● ●

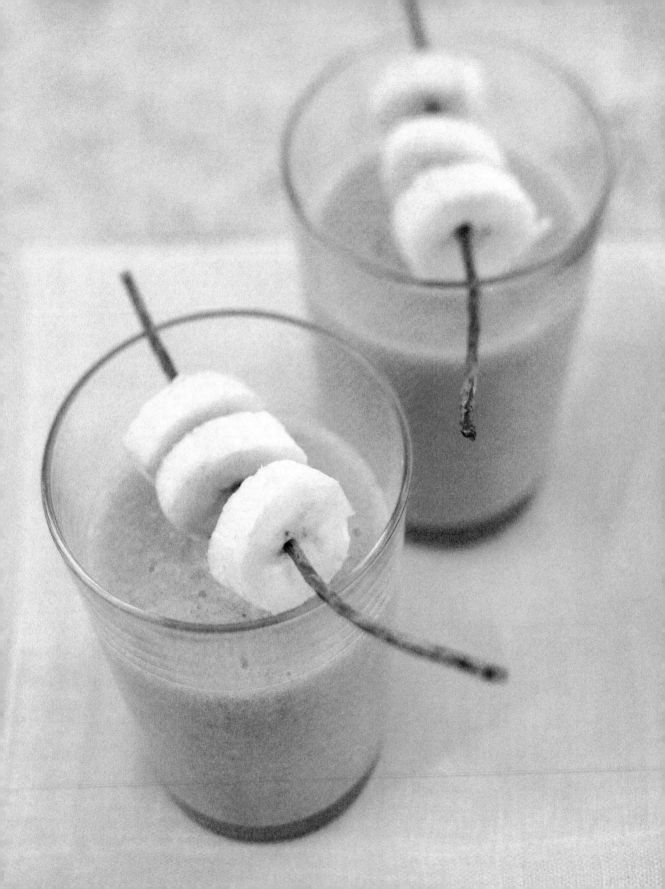

3

SMOOTHIES GALORE

TROPICAL PIÑA COLADA SMOOTHIE

QUICK
& EASY

IMMUNITY
BOOST

THYROID
SUPPORT

KIDNEY
SUPPORT

This is a taste of vacation in a glass, but without the rum. Serve this while relaxing by the pool, or anytime you want to feel like you're on a tropical island.

Recipe Tip You can use either the coconut milk found in the refrigerator section of your market or the kind that is shelf-stable. Do not use canned coconut milk for this recipe, as it's far higher in fat and calories.

½ cup unsweetened coconut milk

2½ cups fresh pineapple chunks
  (or canned unsweetened)

1 cup ice cubes

1. To a blender, add the coconut milk, pineapple, and ice.
2. Blend until smooth.
3. Serve in a tall glass.

Serves 1. Prep time: 2 minutes

PER SERVING: CALORIES: 175 / TOTAL FAT: 3.2G / CARBOHYDRATES: 38.9G / FIBER: 3.8G / PROTEIN: 1.7G

QUICK
& EASY

IMMUNITY
BOOST

THYROID
SUPPORT

KIDNEY
SUPPORT

BANANA NUT BREAD SMOOTHIE

Fresh vanilla beans add a nice flavor without the added sugar or alcohol found in vanilla extract. They're available in the spice section of many grocery stores. To prepare them, use a sharp knife to slice open the pod lengthwise and scrape the contents of the pod (the black seeds) into your recipe.

Recipe Tip Use a frozen banana and skip the ice cubes for a creamier treat. Or, use almond milk or coconut milk and skip the water.

1 cup filtered water

1 medium banana, peeled

¼ cup raw almonds

½ teaspoon cinnamon

¼ teaspoon nutmeg

1 whole vanilla bean, split lengthwise
   and seeds scraped out

½ cup ice cubes

1. To a blender, add the water, banana, almonds, cinnamon, nutmeg, vanilla bean seeds, and ice.
2. Blend until smooth.
3. Serve in a tall glass.

Serves 1. Prep time: 2 minutes

PER SERVING: CALORIES: 254 / TOTAL FAT: 12.1G / CARBOHYDRATES: 33.4G / FIBER: 7.2G / PROTEIN: 6.3G

ORANGE YOU GLAD IT'S HEALTHY SMOOTHIE

This smoothie will remind you of that delicious orange frozen treat you can often get at the mall. Without the sugar and dairy, you can enjoy this whipped smoothie anytime and still stay on your diet plan. If your orange juice isn't that sweet, you can add a packet of stevia. Like all the smoothies in this chapter, be sure to drink it right away or the ingredients will start to separate.

Recipe Tip If freshly squeezed orange juice isn't available, you can use the kind in a carton. Just make sure it's organic and doesn't have any added sugar. Avoid the kind that comes from concentrate that is rehydrated.

6 ounces freshly squeezed orange juice

1 ounce unsweetened coconut milk

1 medium frozen banana, cut into chunks

1 vanilla bean, split lengthwise and seeds scraped out

1 packet stevia (optional)

1. In a blender, add the orange juice, coconut milk, banana, vanilla bean seeds, and stevia (if using).
2. Process until smooth.
3. Serve in a tall glass.

Serves 1. Prep time: 2 minutes

PER SERVING: CALORIES: 182 / TOTAL FAT: 0.3G / CARBOHYDRATES: 44G / FIBER: 3.8G / PROTEIN: 2.3G

QUICK
& EASY

IMMUNITY
BOOST

THYROID
SUPPORT

KIDNEY
SUPPORT

MANGO, PAPAYA, RASPBERRY SMOOTHIE

Mango is one fruit that freezes very well. This is a good thing, as you can have a tropical fruit smoothie any time of year. Papayas are incredibly high in vitamin C, which make them great for fighting off colds or other infections (or avoiding scurvy if you're a pirate). For an added flair, layer the different fruits individually in your glass, rather than blending them all together.

Recipe Tip You can find frozen mango alongside other frozen fruits in your local market. Add water, as needed, if the smoothie is too thick after it is blended.

¼ cup raspberries

¾ cup frozen mango pieces

½ medium papaya, seeds removed
and chopped

1. In a blender, add the raspberries, mango, and papaya.
2. Process until smooth.
3. Serve in a tall glass.

Serves 1. Prep time: 2 minutes

PER SERVING: CALORIES: 153 / TOTAL FAT: 0.06G / CARBOHYDRATES: 39.7G / FIBER: 6.7G / PROTEIN: 2.1G

CHERRY–CHOCOLATE SMOOTHIE

QUICK
& EASY

IMMUNITY
BOOST

THYROID
SUPPORT

KIDNEY
SUPPORT

Although regular cocoa powder is on the "No Go" list when following the Alkaline Diet, Dutch-processed cocoa powder (in limited quantities) is okay since the way it's processed creates an alkalizing effect. Regular cocoa powder has a pH of 5.1 to 5.4; processed cocoa powder is more neutral, with a pH of 6.8 to 8.1. And, because all cocoa powder is so strong, just a touch will give you that chocolate flavor without adding extra acid to your recipe.

Recipe Tip Several popular chocolate brands make a Dutch-processed cocoa, so look for it in your local market, or check the Resources section to buy it online.

½ cup frozen dark cherries

¾ cup filtered water

1 teaspoon Dutch-processed cocoa powder

1 packet stevia (optional)

1. In a blender, add the cherries, water, cocoa powder, and stevia (if using).
2. Process until smooth.
3. Serve in a tall glass.

Serves 1. Prep time: 2 minutes

PER SERVING: CALORIES: 60 / TOTAL FAT: 0.6G / CARBOHYDRATES: 13.2G / FIBER: 1.8G / PROTEIN: 0.5G

QUICK
& EASY

IMMUNITY
BOOST

THYROID
SUPPORT

KIDNEY
SUPPORT

BETTER-THAN-A-COFFEEHOUSE PUMPKIN DRINK

One of the first signs of fall is the appearance of pumpkin spice everything. With this recipe, you can have your ice-blended pumpkin tradition, without the acid-producing ingredients of dairy, sugar, and coffee. Instead, you're replacing them with fiber, antioxidants, minerals, and vitamins. And it's so delicious you won't even miss the bad stuff.

Recipe Tip Make sure you use pumpkin purée (pure pumpkin) and not "pumpkin pie filling." The pie filling is filled with sugar and dairy.

½ cup pumpkin purée

1 banana, frozen

1 cup unsweetened coconut milk

1 vanilla bean, split lengthwise and seeds scraped out

¼ teaspoon cinnamon

⅛ teaspoon nutmeg

⅛ teaspoon allspice

½ cup ice cubes

1. In a blender, add the pumpkin, banana, coconut milk, vanilla bean seeds, cinnamon, nutmeg, allspice, and ice.
2. Process until smooth.
3. Serve in a tall glass.

Serves 1. Prep time: 2 minutes

PER SERVING: CALORIES: 240 / TOTAL FAT: 5.5G / CARBOHYDRATES: 47.6G / FIBER: 7.6G / PROTEIN: 3.6G

BASIC GREEN SMOOTHIE

QUICK
& EASY

IMMUNITY
BOOST

THYROID
SUPPORT

KIDNEY
SUPPORT

There is no need to be scared of the green smoothie. It can really be delicious if you follow the basic formula. To make an easy, healthy, and tasty green smoothie, blend together one cup of a leafy green vegetable, plus one cup of a liquid base, plus one cup of fruit. Try this one for starters.

Recipe Tip Feel free to use whatever kind of fruit you prefer instead of peaches here. Just avoid blueberries, as they're on the "No Go" list.

1 cup spinach

1 cup unsweetened coconut milk

1 cup frozen sliced peaches

1. In a blender, add the spinach, coconut milk, and peaches.
2. Process until smooth.
3. Serve in a tall glass.

Serves 1. Prep time: 2 minutes

PER SERVING: CALORIES: 230 / TOTAL FAT: 6G / CARBOHYDRATES: 43.5G / FIBER: 5.8G / PROTEIN: 4.9G

QUICK
& EASY

IMMUNITY
BOOST

THYROID
SUPPORT

KIDNEY
SUPPORT

MORE-THAN-A-MOJITO SMOOTHIE

Although citrus fruit is acidic, once your body processes it, the result is an alkalizing effect. So, the lime juice in this recipe adds flavor but not acid. This drink is a great alternative to a cocktail. It's packed with nutrition instead of empty calories.

Recipe Tip You can substitute key limes for a sweeter taste. These tiny limes are less tart than regular limes.

1 cup spinach

1 cup unsweetened coconut water

2 cups pineapple

2 tablespoons fresh mint leaves

Juice of ½ lime

1. In a blender, add the spinach, coconut water, pineapple, mint leaves, and lime juice.
2. Process until smooth.
3. Serve in a tall glass.

Serves 1. Prep time: 2 minutes

PER SERVING: CALORIES: 241 / TOTAL FAT: 1.5G / CARBOHYDRATES: 60.4G / FIBER: 5.3G / PROTEIN: 2.6G

LIQUID GUACAMOLE

QUICK
& EASY

IMMUNITY
BOOST

KIDNEY
SUPPORT

The name of this recipe might take a little getting used to, but it is delicious! An avocado actually adds a delicious smooth texture that you cannot get from anything else. Try this as a filling appetizer before a Mexican-inspired (alkaline-friendly, of course) main meal.

Recipe Tip If you're on the Thyroid-Support Plan, don't use this recipe. In fact, avoid any recipes in the book that contain tomatoes or tomato products.

½ avocado

1 cup spinach

¼ cup cilantro

1 cup fresh tomato juice

Pinch garlic powder

Pinch sea salt

Pinch cayenne pepper

½ cup cherry tomatoes

½ cup diced cucumber

1. In a blender, add the avocado, spinach, cilantro, tomato juice, garlic powder, salt, and cayenne.
2. Blend until smooth.
3. Add the cherry tomatoes and cucumber, and blend until small chunks remain.
4. Serve in a tall glass.

Serves 1. Prep time: 2 minutes

PER SERVING: CALORIES: 274 / TOTAL FAT: 20.1G / CARBOHYDRATES: 24.8G / FIBER: 9.5G / PROTEIN: 5.6G

QUICK
& EASY

IMMUNITY
BOOST

THYROID
SUPPORT

KIDNEY
SUPPORT

THE "CAN THIS BE KALE?" SMOOTHIE

No chapter on smoothies is complete without a kale recipe or two. Many people don't like kale because of its bitter taste and the fact that it looks like something used to line a salad bar. The key to using kale is to pair it with very sweet fruits. Of course, if you love kale, then use more!

Recipe Tip Stevia is an all-natural sweetener that comes from the leaf of the stevia plant. Make sure the kind you choose isn't mixed with lactose, which is a dairy product.

½ cup kale

1 medium banana, extra ripe

1 cup fresh pineapple juice

½ cup ice cubes

1 packet stevia (optional)

1. In a blender, place the kale, banana, pineapple juice, ice, and stevia (if using).
2. Process until smooth.
3. Serve in a tall glass.

Serves 1. Prep time: 2 minutes

PER SERVING: CALORIES: 254 / TOTAL FAT: 0.03G / CARBOHYDRATES: 62.5G / FIBER: 4.5G / PROTEIN: 3.1G

ORANGE, PEACH, KALE SMOOTHIE

QUICK
& EASY

IMMUNITY
BOOST

THYROID
SUPPORT

KIDNEY
SUPPORT

The most time-consuming part of this delicious recipe is peeling the orange. Since that doesn't exactly take long, this is a great recipe for those busy mornings when you are rushing out the door and want to grab something quickly. For an even faster smoothie, use frozen peaches. Just blend and go!

Recipe Tip If you can't find a fresh peach, frozen will do. If the only peaches available are canned, drain and rinse before using.

1 orange, peeled and seeded

1 medium peach, peeled and sliced

1 cup chopped kale

8 ounces filtered water

1. In a blender, place the orange, peach, kale, and water.
2. Process until smooth.
3. Serve in a tall glass.

Serves 1. Prep time: 10 minutes

PER SERVING: CALORIES: 158 / TOTAL FAT: 0.05G / CARBOHYDRATES: 38G / FIBER: 6.9G / PROTEIN: 4.6G

QUICK
& EASY

IMMUNITY
BOOST

THYROID
SUPPORT

KIDNEY
SUPPORT

CUCUMBER SOUP IN A CUP

This cool cucumber smoothie is perfect for those hot days when you don't want to heat up the kitchen. The combination of avocado and cucumber is classic. This savory smoothie is full of nutrition and taste—and it's alkaline, too!

Recipe Tip Add a dash of cayenne pepper for a touch of heat.

1 cup peeled and diced cucumber

½ avocado

½ cup cold water

½ cup ice cubes

Pinch garlic powder

Pinch sea salt

1. In a blender, add the cucumber, avocado, water, ice, garlic powder, and sea salt.
2. Process until desired consistency.
3. Serve in a tall glass.

Serves 1. Prep time: 5 minutes

PER SERVING: CALORIES: 221 / TOTAL FAT: 19.7G / CARBOHYDRATES: 12.4G /
FIBER: 7.2G / PROTEIN: 2.6G

GAZPACHO SMOOTHIE

QUICK
& EASY

IMMUNITY
BOOST

KIDNEY
SUPPORT

Gazpacho is a Spanish soup traditionally made with raw vegetables and served cold. That sounds like a great base for a smoothie! Leave the "soup" a little chunky if you wish, or blend it completely. Serve with a celery stalk as a stirrer for fun.

Recipe Tip Because this is a cold smoothie, you can use frozen red bell peppers.

½ carrot, peeled and chopped

½ celery stalk, chopped

¼ onion, chopped

1 medium tomato, chopped

2 cups spinach

½ red bell pepper, seeded and chopped

½ cucumber, peeled and chopped

¼ cup fresh cilantro, stemmed

¼ teaspoon cumin

¼ teaspoon garlic powder

Pinch sea salt

Fresh tomato juice, as needed

1. In a blender, place the carrot, celery, onion, tomato, spinach, red bell pepper, cucumber, cilantro, cumin, garlic powder, and salt.
2. Pulse until the desired consistency.
3. If the mixture is too thick, slowly add the tomato juice until you have the desired consistency.
4. Serve in a tall glass.

Serves 1. Prep time: 15 minutes

PER SERVING: CALORIES: 102 / TOTAL FAT: 0.8G / CARBOHYDRATES: 21.7G / FIBER: 6.3G / PROTEIN: 4.9G

QUICK
& EASY

IMMUNITY
BOOST

THYROID
SUPPORT

KIDNEY
SUPPORT

SPARKLING LIME–ASIAN PEAR GREEN SMOOTHIE

Although spinach and kale are the most popular greens for smoothies, this recipe uses Chinese cabbage for a twist. If you can't find Asian pears, any type of pear will work. Fresh ginger is best, but powdered will work as well. Also, remember that when blending sparkling water, it will expand, so be sure to cover the top of the blender to avoid a mess.

Recipe Tip If you can't find lime-flavored sparkling water, use plain and add a squeeze or two of fresh lime juice.

1 cup unsweetened, lime-flavored
  sparkling water
1 Asian pear, peeled and sliced
½ cup Chinese cabbage

1 teaspoon grated fresh ginger
1 packet stevia
½ cup ice cubes

1. In the blender, place the sparkling water, pear, cabbage, ginger, stevia, and ice.
2. Carefully process, covered, until blended.
3. Serve in a tall glass.

Serves 1. Prep time: 5 minutes

PER SERVING: CALORIES: 85 / TOTAL FAT: 0.2G / CARBOHYDRATES: 22.3G / FIBER: 4.6G / PROTEIN: 1G

WARM GINGER, GARLIC, LEMON SMOOTHIE

QUICK
& EASY

IMMUNITY
BOOST

THYROID
SUPPORT

KIDNEY
SUPPORT

Who says a smoothie has to be cold? This is a great, healing smoothie for those days when you're feeling a little off or are fighting an illness. The raw garlic can be a bit sharp, but it contains healthful properties that powdered garlic doesn't. Add some cayenne pepper if you wish to spice things up even more.

Recipe Tip Keep a container of reconstituted lemon juice in your refrigerator. It's perfect for times when you don't have fresh lemons on hand.

1 cup warm water

Juice of 1 lemon

¼ teaspoon grated fresh ginger

1 garlic clove, peeled

½ teaspoon sesame oil

¼ teaspoon sea salt

1. In a blender, add the water, lemon juice, ginger, garlic, sesame oil, and salt.
2. Pulse until the desired consistency.
3. Serve in a tall glass.

Serves 1. Prep time: 2 minutes

PER SERVING: CALORIES: 26 / TOTAL FAT: 2.3G / CARBOHYDRATES: 1.3G / PROTEIN: 0.2G

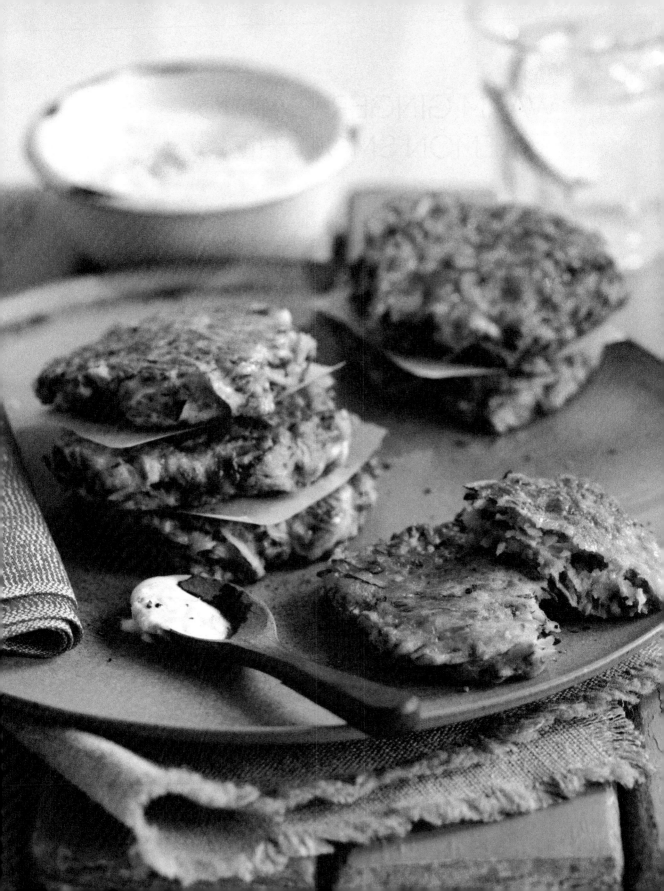

4

BALANCED BREAKFASTS

GOOD MORNING POPEYE

QUICK
& EASY

IMMUNITY
BOOST

THYROID
SUPPORT

KIDNEY
SUPPORT

This dish is easy to prepare the night before (up until the cooking step) so you can cut down on prep time in the morning. Since it only takes about 10 minutes of actual cooking time, you can have a home-cooked breakfast any day of the week! For even quicker preparation, you can pop the sweet potatoes in the microwave for two to three minutes to par-cook. Or, if you prefer, combine the ingredients in a baking dish and bake at 350°F for 30 minutes while getting dressed and ready to leave the house.

Recipe Tip Keep a bag of chopped onions in your freezer so you can just measure out what you need. You don't even need to defrost them; just add them to the pan frozen.

1 tablespoon coconut oil

2 medium sweet potatoes, peeled and cubed

1 medium sweet onion, chopped

1 red bell pepper, cored, seeded, and chopped

¼ cup sliced mushrooms, any type

2 garlic cloves, chopped

4 cups spinach

1 teaspoon onion powder

1 teaspoon garlic powder

½ teaspoon Bouquet Garni herb blend, or other dried herbs such as rosemary or sage

½ teaspoon sea salt

1. In a medium bowl, combine the oil, sweet potatoes, onion, red bell pepper, mushrooms, garlic, spinach, onion powder, garlic powder, Bouquet Garni, and salt. Toss until the oil and seasonings are distributed evenly on the vegetables.
2. Heat a nonstick frying pan over medium heat and add the contents of the bowl. Cook the vegetables, stirring, for 10 minutes, or until tender.
3. Divide into two portions and serve.

Serves 2. Prep time: 5 minutes. Cook time: 10 minutes

PER SERVING (½ FINISHED RECIPE): CALORIES: 181 / TOTAL FAT: 1.5G / CARBOHYDRATES: 37.8G / FIBER: 8.1G / PROTEIN: 5.6G

GARDEN PANCAKES

QUICK
& EASY

IMMUNITY
BOOST

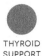

THYROID
SUPPORT

KIDNEY
SUPPORT

Feel free to substitute any vegetables you like in this recipe. Just be sure to choose ones that aren't too high in water content (like tomatoes) or the pancakes will fall apart. Since these aren't bound with egg, be very careful when you flip them over. Serve these savory pancakes with salsa instead of syrup.

Recipe Tip You can make your own almond flour by grinding raw almonds in a food processor.

1 medium zucchini, roughly chopped

1 carrot, peeled and roughly chopped

1 yellow squash, roughly chopped

½ small onion, grated

4 scallions

¼ cup almond flour

1 teaspoon sea salt

½ teaspoon garlic powder

¼ cup filtered water, as needed

Cooking spray for greasing the pan

1. Place the zucchini, carrot, yellow squash, onion, scallions, almond flour, salt, and garlic powder in a food processor. Pulse until blended.
2. Add only enough water to make the mixture moist, not runny. The batter will be fairly thick.
3. Spray a large nonstick skillet or griddle with cooking spray. Set the skillet over medium-high heat.
4. When the oil is hot, use an ice cream scoop or ¼-cup measure to drop the batter into the skillet. With a fork, spread the batter evenly, pressing down on the pancakes. Cook, turning once, until nicely browned on both sides, about 5 minutes total.
5. Serve hot or at room temperature.

Serves 2. Prep time: 5 minutes. Cook time: 5 minutes

PER SERVING (3 PANCAKES): CALORIES: 254 / TOTAL FAT: 12.1G / CARBOHYDRATES: 33.4G / FIBER: 7.2G / PROTEIN: 6.3G

TROPICAL GRANOLA

QUICK
& EASY

IMMUNITY
BOOST

THYROID
SUPPORT

KIDNEY
SUPPORT

There is no need for sugary, processed commercial granola when you can make it healthy at home in less time than it takes to go to the market. This version does not have the traditional oats or sugar, but is filled with naturally sweet and crunchy items. Be sure to avoid using regular shredded coconut as it has a lot of sugar. You can find flaked unsweetened coconut at many regular markets and most health food stores.

Recipe Tip This granola will keep in an airtight container for a week or so. Or make an extra batch, and freeze it to have on hand for months!

1 cup flaked unsweetened coconut

1 cup slivered almonds

½ cup flaxseed

½ cup raisins

½ teaspoon cinnamon

¼ teaspoon ginger

¼ teaspoon nutmeg

¼ teaspoon sea salt

1 vanilla bean, split lengthwise and seeds scraped out

¼ cup coconut oil

½ cup unsweetened dried pineapple tidbits

1. Preheat the oven to 350°F.
2. In a medium bowl, combine the coconut, almonds, flaxseed, raisins, cinnamon, ginger, nutmeg, salt, vanilla bean seeds, and coconut oil. Toss until well combined.
3. Spread the mixture evenly on a baking sheet and place it into the preheated oven. Bake for 15 minutes, stirring occasionally, until golden brown.
4. Remove from the oven and cool, without stirring.
5. Once cooled, stir in the pineapple tidbits.
6. Store in an airtight container.

Serves 4. Prep time: 2 minutes. Cook time: 15 minutes

PER SERVING (SCANT 1 CUP): CALORIES: 182 / TOTAL FAT: 0.3G / CARBOHYDRATES: 44G / FIBER: 3.8G / PROTEIN: 2.3G

QUICK
& EASY

IMMUNITY
BOOST

THYROID
SUPPORT

KIDNEY
SUPPORT

SUMMER FRUIT SALAD WITH LIME AND MINT

There are few things better than sitting outside on a beautiful morning enjoying a cool fruit salad. Make this the night before so the mint has time to mingle with the fruits. And, as always, feel free to substitute any fruits you prefer. Just avoid blueberries, as they're on the "No Go" list.

Recipe Tip If you don't have time to make this the night before, you can make it and serve it right away. It's delicious either way.

¼ cup grapes

¼ cup peeled and diced apple

¼ cup bite-size watermelon pieces

¼ cup bite-size honeydew melon pieces

¼ cup bite-size cantaloupe pieces

¼ cup tangerine slices

¼ cup peeled and diced peaches

¼ cup strawberries

2 tablespoons chopped fresh mint

2 tablespoons freshly squeezed lemon juice

1. In a medium bowl, combine the grapes, apple, watermelon, honeydew, cantaloupe, tangerine, peaches, and strawberries.
2. Add the mint and lemon juice. Mix well to combine. Cover and refrigerate overnight.
3. Spoon into four bowls, and serve chilled.

Serves 4. Prep time: 10 minutes

PER SERVING (½ CUP): CALORIES: 32 / TOTAL FAT: 0.02G / CARBOHYDRATES: 7.8G / FIBER: 0.09G / PROTEIN: 0.6G

WINTER FRUIT COMPOTE WITH FIGS AND GINGER

This recipe is the winter equivalent of a summer fruit salad. It's basically a warm fruit stew that is comforting and healthy on a cold winter morning. Feel free to add different fruits you prefer. This is also great for dessert.

Recipe Tip This is also delicious served cold. Top it with Coconut Whipped Cream (page 202) for a delicious and healthy dessert.

2 small tangerines, peeled and sectioned

1 apple, peeled, cored, and diced

½ cup figs, stemmed and quartered

½ cup dried plums (prunes), halved

¼ cup dark cherries

1 cup filtered water

1 vanilla bean, split lengthwise and seeds scraped out

1 teaspoon grated fresh ginger

½ teaspoon cinnamon

½ teaspoon cloves

1 packet stevia (optional)

1. In a medium saucepan, combine the tangerines, apple, figs, dried plums, cherries, water, vanilla bean seeds, ginger, cinnamon, cloves, and stevia (if using).
2. Bring to a simmer over medium heat and cook, stirring occasionally, for 10 minutes, or until the fruit is tender but not too soft. Remove from the heat.
3. Let stand for 30 minutes to meld the flavors.
4. Reheat if necessary, spoon into four bowls and serve warm.

Serves 4. Prep time: 10 minutes. Cook time: 10 minutes

PER SERVING (1 CUP): CALORIES: 102 / TOTAL FAT: 0.4G / CARBOHYDRATES: 26G / FIBER: 4.2G / PROTEIN: 1G

ALL–AMERICAN APPLE PIE

QUICK
& EASY

IMMUNITY
BOOST

THYROID
SUPPORT

KIDNEY
SUPPORT

Imagine the looks on your kids' faces when you tell them they can have apple pie for breakfast. Of course, this apple pie is healthy! Since this is a breakfast recipe, this version is crustless. But if you want to make it for dessert, use the recipe for All-Purpose Pie Crust (page 181) and top with some Coconut Ice Cream (page 182).

Recipe Tip You can use any kind of apples for this pie. Generally speaking, green apples keep their shape better than other kinds when cooked. But use your favorite here and enjoy.

4 Golden Delicious apples, peeled, cored, and sliced

½ cup freshly squeezed orange juice

1 vanilla bean, split lengthwise and seeds scraped out

¼ teaspoon cinnamon

Unsweetened coconut milk, as needed (optional)

1. In a large bowl, toss the apples with the orange juice, vanilla bean seeds, and cinnamon.
2. In a medium skillet set over medium heat, add the fruit mixture. Cook for 10 minutes, or until the apples are soft and caramelized.
3. Divide the mixture among four serving dishes, and serve warm.
4. Top with coconut milk (if using).

Serves 4. Prep time: 10 minutes. Cook time: 10 minutes

PER SERVING (1 CUP): CALORIES: 109 / TOTAL FAT: 0.1G / CARBOHYDRATES: 28.5G / FIBER: 4.5G / PROTEIN: 0.2G

BABY POTATO HOME FRIES

Who needs the high-fat, high-sodium restaurant version of home fries? Instead, this healthy version uses baby white potatoes and a nonstick pan to give you all the flavor without the acid-producing side effects. If you have leftovers, you can chill them and make a potato salad. It's breakfast or lunch!

Recipe Tip You can also use small red potatoes for this recipe. It's best to avoid the brown russet potatoes typically used for baking as they contain a lot of starch.

4 medium baby white potatoes

2 ounces vegetable broth

½ sweet white onion, chopped

1 red bell pepper, seeded and diced

½ cup sliced mushrooms

1 teaspoon sea salt

1 teaspoon garlic powder

1. In a medium microwave-safe bowl, microwave the potatoes for 4 minutes, or until soft. Let cool.
2. In a large nonstick skillet set over medium heat, add the broth, onion, and red bell pepper. Sauté the vegetables for about 5 minutes, or until soft.
3. While the onion and peppers cook, cut the potatoes into quarters.
4. Add the potatoes, mushrooms, salt, and garlic powder to the skillet. Stir to combine. Cook for about 10 minutes, or until the potatoes are crisp.
5. Serve warm.

Serves 2. Prep time: 5 minutes. Cook time: 20 minutes

PER SERVING (1 CUP): CALORIES: 337 / TOTAL FAT: 0.8G / CARBOHYDRATES: 74.8G / FIBER: 12.4G / PROTEIN: 9.3G

BREAKFAST FAJITAS

QUICK
& EASY

IMMUNITY
BOOST

KIDNEY
SUPPORT

This restaurant staple can easily be adapted as a fantastic breakfast meal. It's a great way to load up on healthy veggies and fill your belly to start your day. Wrap these fajitas in lettuce leaves, if you wish, but they are outstanding just eaten hot from the skillet with a fork.

Recipe Tip There is a source link in the Resources section for coconut-flour tortillas. Wrap one of those around these fajitas for a filling breakfast.

Cooking spray

1 bell pepper, any color, cored, seeded, and sliced

1 sweet onion, such as Vidalia, chopped

1 cup cooked broccoli florets

½ cup sliced mushrooms

1 cup cherry tomatoes, halved if large

½ cup sliced zucchini, or other squash

2 garlic cloves, peeled and chopped

1 jalapeño, chopped (optional)

1 teaspoon sea salt

½ teaspoon cumin

2 tablespoons fresh cilantro

Juice of ½ lime

Salsa Fresca (page 198), for serving

1. Spray a large nonstick skillet with cooking spray and place it over medium heat.
2. Add the bell pepper, onion, broccoli, mushrooms, tomatoes, zucchini, garlic, and jalapeño (if using). Cook, stirring, for about 7 minutes, or until the desired level of tenderness.
3. Stir in the salt, cumin, and cilantro. Cook, stirring, for 3 minutes more.
4. Remove from heat and add the lime juice.
5. Divide between two plates and serve with Salsa Fresca.

Serves 2. Prep time: 5 minutes. Cook time: 10 minutes

PER SERVING (½ FINISHED RECIPE): CALORIES: 86 / TOTAL FAT: 0.07G /

CARBOHYDRATES: 17.4G / FIBER: 5.1G / PROTEIN: 4.1G

GRANDMA'S BAKED GRAPEFRUIT

QUICK
& EASY

IMMUNITY
BOOST

THYROID
SUPPORT

KIDNEY
SUPPORT

Grapefruit is great at any temperature, but it is especially good baked. This vitamin C-rich fruit is packed with fiber and nutrition. When baked, it's typically topped with brown sugar or maple syrup, but this version uses grated coconut instead. Make this warming breakfast on a chilly day.

Recipe Tip Ruby Red is a variety of grapefruit that tends to be sweeter than other kinds. If you're not a big grapefruit fan, try Ruby Red first.

1 grapefruit, halved
2 tablespoons grated unsweetened coconut

1. Preheat the oven to 350°F.
2. Place the grapefruit halves on a foil-lined baking pan. Top each half with 1 tablespoon of coconut.
3. Place the pan in the preheated oven and bake for 15 minutes, or until the coconut is browned.
4. Serve the grapefruit halves on a plate and eat with a spoon.

Serves 1. Prep time: 15 minutes. Cook time: 15 minutes

PER SERVING: CALORIES: 86 / TOTAL FAT: 0.07G / CARBOHYDRATES: 11.9G / FIBER: 2.3G / PROTEIN: 1.2G

BREAKFAST PARFAIT

QUICK
& EASY

IMMUNITY
BOOST

THYROID
SUPPORT

KIDNEY
SUPPORT

This version of a fruit parfait is so easy to make you're going to wonder why you never made it before. Instead of yogurt or whipped cream, this recipe calls for Coconut Whipped Cream (page 202).

Recipe Tip Feel free to swap in any fruits you like. Get bold and layer in things like pumpkin or sweet potato!

¼ cup sliced strawberries

¼ cup blackberries

¼ cup sliced raspberries

¼ cup sliced peaches

1 cup Coconut Whipped Cream (page 202)

1. In a large clear glass, place 2 tablespoons strawberries and top with 2 tablespoons whipped cream. Add 2 tablespoons blackberries and another 2 tablespoons whipped cream. Continue with 2 tablespoons raspberries and 2 tablespoons whipped cream. Finish with 2 tablespoons peaches and 2 tablespoons whipped cream.
2. Repeat with the remaining ingredients in a second glass.
3. Serve immediately.

Serves 2. Prep time: 10 minutes

PER SERVING (½ CUP FRUIT WITH ½ CUP COCONUT WHIPPED CREAM): CALORIES: 120 / TOTAL FAT: 10G / CARBOHYDRATES: 4G / FIBER: 6.3G / PROTEIN: 1.7G

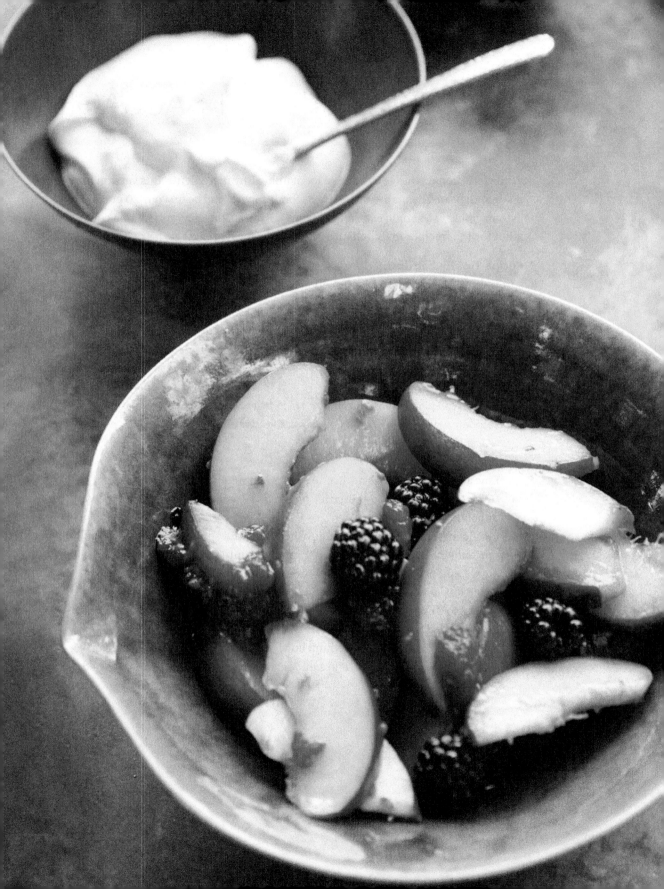

HEARTY BREAKFAST SAUSAGE

While traditional sausage contains a lot of unhealthy ingredients, this version is made with beans. Beans are one of those foods that should be on your 20 percent list—meaning you should eat them sparingly. Even so, this is a protein-rich complement to other recipes in this chapter. And, in the form of sausage, it's delicious, too!

Recipe Tip You can dry fry these sausage patties by cooking them in a nonstick pan sprayed with cooking spray. Fry for about 5 minutes per side.

2 garlic cloves

1 small onion, quartered

1 carrot, peeled and cut into large chunks

½ teaspoon fennel seeds

Water, as needed

1 (15-ounce) can pinto beans, drained

1 tablespoon almond flour or almond meal

1 tablespoon nutritional yeast

1 teaspoon smoked paprika

½ teaspoon dried oregano (1 teaspoon fresh)

½ teaspoon dried sage (1 teaspoon fresh)

½ teaspoon dried basil (1 teaspoon fresh)

½ teaspoon dried thyme (1 teaspoon fresh)

½ teaspoon sea salt

1. Preheat the oven to 400°F.
2. Line a baking sheet with a silicone mat or parchment paper.
3. In a food processor, add the garlic, onion, and carrot. Chop until fine, or chop by hand.
4. Place a medium skillet over medium heat. Add the onion-carrot mixture, and the fennel seeds. Cook for about 4 minutes or until the vegetables are soft, adding water if needed. Remove from the heat and cool.
5. In the food processor, add the pinto beans and pulse until roughly chopped, but not to a paste. Add the onion-carrot mixture to the processor, and process until blended.
6. Transfer the contents to a medium bowl. Add the almond flour, yeast, paprika, oregano, sage, basil, thyme, and salt. Mix until the ingredients are combined.

7. Measure ¼ cup of sausage and shape into a patty by hand. Carefully place each patty onto the prepared pan. Continue with the remaining sausage.
8. Bake for 25 to 30 minutes, until crispy on the outside but still moist on the inside.
9. Remove from the oven and cool for a few minutes before serving.

Serves 9. Prep time: 20 minutes. Cook time: 35 minutes

PER SERVING (1 PATTY): CALORIES: 69 / TOTAL FAT: 1.7G / CARBOHYDRATES: 10.7G / FIBER: 3G / PROTEIN: 3.5G

SWEET POTATO WAFFLES WITH APPLESAUCE

QUICK & EASY

IMMUNITY BOOST

THYROID SUPPORT

KIDNEY SUPPORT

This recipe might just become your new Sunday morning tradition. These waffles (or pancakes, if you don't have a waffle iron) are so healthy and delicious you won't even miss the acid-producing buttermilk ones you're used to eating. Be careful when removing them from the waffle iron, as they are extremely moist and fragile. If one does fall apart, eat it and call it your "chef's bonus."

Recipe Tip If you don't have applesauce, serve these with Apple Butter (page 203).

1¼ cups almond flour

2 teaspoons baking powder

½ teaspoon sea salt

Dash nutmeg

Dash cinnamon

⅓ cup coconut oil

1½ cups unsweetened coconut milk

1 cup mashed sweet potato

Cooking spray

1 cup unsweetened applesauce

1. Preheat the waffle iron.
2. In a large bowl, combine the almond flour, baking powder, salt, nutmeg, and cinnamon.
3. In a medium bowl, whisk together the coconut oil and coconut milk until combined.
4. Transfer the liquid ingredients to the bowl with the dry ingredients. Whisk until combined.
5. Gently fold the sweet potatoes into the batter, being careful not to over mix.
6. Spray the waffle iron with cooking spray before making each waffle.
7. Make the waffles according to the directions indicated on the waffle iron.
8. Serve each waffle with ¼ cup of applesauce.

Serves 4. Prep time: 15 minutes. Cook time: 5 to 7 minutes

PER SERVING (1 WAFFLE WITH ¼ CUP APPLESAUCE): CALORIES: 547 / TOTAL FAT: 25G / CARBOHYDRATES: 38G / FIBER: 16.9G / PROTEIN: 14.6G

SPAGHETTI SQUASH HASH BROWNS

QUICK
& EASY

IMMUNITY
BOOST

THYROID
SUPPORT

KIDNEY
SUPPORT

Who needs the high-fat, acid-producing restaurant hash browns when you can make these delicious and nutritious ones at home? This recipe calls for cooked spaghetti squash, so the day before you make these, just pop a spaghetti squash in the oven, and roast it (see note below). This way, the recipe takes only a few minutes to prepare. Serve with Hearty Breakfast Sausage (page 70) and Homemade Ketchup (page 197). Just remember to skip the ketchup if you're following the Thyroid-Support Plan.

Recipe Tip Make sure you squeeze as much moisture as you can from the spaghetti squash so it will crisp.

2 cups cooked spaghetti squash

½ cup finely chopped onion

1 teaspoon garlic powder

½ teaspoon sea salt

Cooking spray

1. Using paper towel, squeeze any excess moisture from the spaghetti squash. Place the squash in a medium bowl. Add the onion, garlic powder, and salt. Mix to combine.
2. Spray a medium nonstick skillet with cooking spray and place it over medium heat.
3. Add the squash mixture to the pan. Cook, untouched, for 5 minutes. With a spatula, flip the hash browns. It's okay if the mixture falls apart. Cook for about 5 minutes more, or until the desired level of crispness.

To roast a spaghetti squash, cut the squash in half lengthwise and scrape out the seeds. Brush each half with 2 tablespoons of coconut oil and season with 1 teaspoon of sea salt. Place the squash halves cut-side up on a baking sheet and roast at 350°F for about 50 minutes, or until fork tender.

Serves 2. Prep time: 2 minutes. Cook time: 10 minutes

PER SERVING (1 CUP): CALORIES: 44 / TOTAL FAT: 0.6G / CARBOHYDRATES: 9.7G / FIBER: 0.6G / PROTEIN: 0.9G

BROWN RICE PORRIDGE

QUICK
& EASY

IMMUNITY
BOOST

THYROID
SUPPORT

KIDNEY
SUPPORT

Brown rice and almond milk replace the white rice and cow's milk traditionally found in this English-inspired breakfast. Feel free to add any fruits you have on hand. Bananas and a little cinnamon will make it hearty; cherries and papaya will make it tropical. Add a touch of coconut milk or almond milk before serving if the porridge is too thick.

Recipe Tip You can buy brown rice cereal in the market. Use it instead of regular brown rice in this recipe to make this alkaline-friendly dish even quicker and easier.

3 cups cooked brown rice

1 cup almond milk

1 packet stevia

1. In a medium saucepan, combine the brown rice and the almond milk. Simmer over medium heat for 5 minutes, stirring constantly, until the mixture is thick and creamy.
2. Remove from heat. Stir in the stevia.
3. Divide among 6 bowls and serve.

Serves 6. Prep time: 5 minutes. Cook time: 5 minutes

PER SERVING (½ CUP PORRIDGE): CALORIES: 236 / TOTAL FAT: 1.8G / CARBOHYDRATES: 48.3G / FIBER: 3.6G / PROTEIN: 7G

PUMPKIN–SPICE QUINOA CASSEROLE

QUICK
& EASY

IMMUNITY
BOOST

THYROID
SUPPORT

KIDNEY
SUPPORT

This hearty casserole can be assembled the night before baking to make morning preparation a snap. Quinoa is a protein powerhouse that adds a nutty flavor. The pumpkin holds its own with tons of beta-carotene and fiber. And using cooked quinoa makes assembly even easier. This breakfast is one that will keep you going all morning long.

Recipe Tip You can actually microwave this dish to make it even faster. Simply pop the mixture into the microwave for 7 minutes on high, or until the pumpkin is set.

Cooking spray

3 cups cooked quinoa

1 (15-ounce) can pumpkin purée

½ cup water

1 vanilla bean, split lengthwise and seeds
  scraped out

1 teaspoon cinnamon

½ teaspoon nutmeg

½ teaspoon ground ginger

¼ teaspoon grated fresh ginger

¼ teaspoon sea salt

1. Preheat the oven to 350°F.
2. Spray a 4-cup casserole dish and set aside.
3. In a medium bowl, stir together the quinoa, pumpkin, water, vanilla bean seeds, cinnamon, nutmeg, ground ginger, fresh ginger, and salt.
4. Transfer the mixture to the prepared casserole dish. Bake for 15 minutes, or until golden and bubbly.

Serves 6. Prep time: 5 minutes. Cook time: 15 minutes

PER SERVING (1 CUP): CALORIES: 26 / TOTAL FAT: 5G / CARBOHYDRATES: 57.1G / FIBER: 7.7G / PROTEIN: 12G

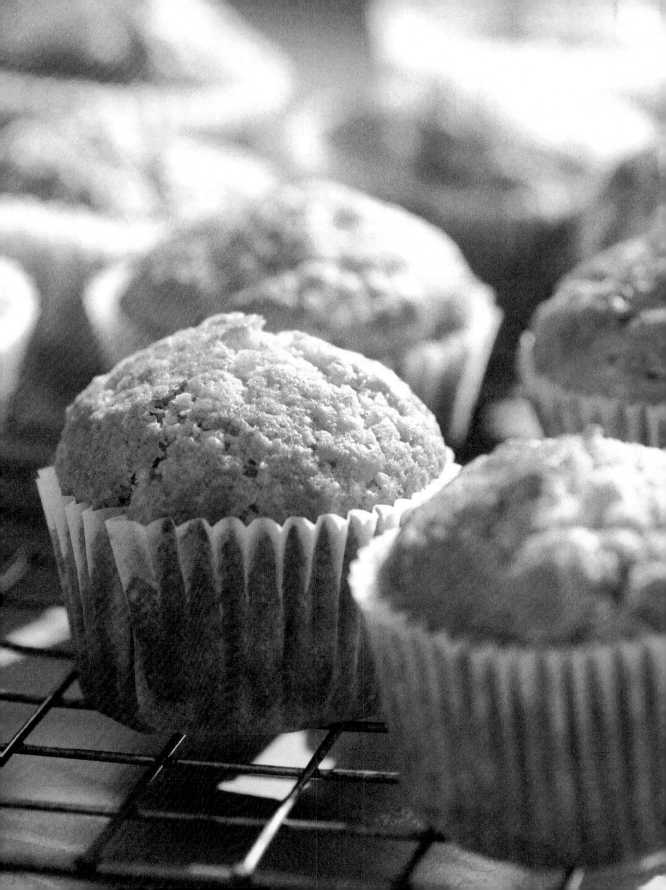

5

BAKED DELIGHTS

BAKED SWEET POTATO AND APPLE

IMMUNITY BOOST

THYROID SUPPORT

KIDNEY SUPPORT

This is a most unusual yet delicious treat. It's great for breakfast or dessert. As an added bonus, your house will fill with the scent of autumn. And, your belly will be filled with nutrition.

Recipe Tip As with the other apple recipes in this book, you can use any type of apple you like. Or, fill the sweet potato with applesauce or Apple Butter (page 203).

1 medium sweet potato

1 medium apple, peeled and diced

½ teaspoon cinnamon

Pinch sea salt

1. Preheat the oven to 350°F.
2. Cut the sweet potato, lengthwise, about 1 inch deep. Spread the potato open and place it in a baking dish.
3. Place the apple inside the sweet potato's opening. Sprinkle the cinnamon and salt on top.
4. Cover with aluminum foil. Place the dish in the preheated oven and bake for 40 minutes, or until the potato is soft.
5. Serve warm.

Serves 1. Prep time: 5 minutes. Cook time: 40 minutes

PER SERVING: CALORIES: 198 / TOTAL FAT: 0.2G / CARBOHYDRATES: 48.7G / FIBER: 8.2G / PROTEIN: 2.3G

QUICK
& EASY

IMMUNITY
BOOST

THYROID
SUPPORT

KIDNEY
SUPPORT

OVEN–BAKED ONION RINGS

These baked onion rings are great as a snack while watching the game, or served as a side dish. Baking them slashes fat and calories. And using almond meal instead of wheat flour makes this recipe alkaline friendly. Serve with Homemade Ketchup (page 197) or Homemade Barbecue Sauce (page 207)—except if you're on the Thyroid-Support Plan, in which case you should avoid foods or condiments containing tomato products.

Recipe Tip For a sweeter onion ring, choose a sweet onion like Vidalia or Maui.

Cooking spray

⅔ cup almond meal

1 teaspoon garlic powder

1 teaspoon onion powder

½ teaspoon paprika

½ teaspoon sea salt

½ cup almond milk

1 large onion, sliced into ¼-inch-thick slices

1. Preheat the oven to 425°F.
2. Spray a baking sheet with cooking spray.
3. On a plate, mix together the almond meal, garlic powder, onion powder, paprika, and sea salt.
4. Pour the almond milk into a medium bowl.
5. Dip one onion slice into the milk. Then dredge it in the seasoned almond meal and place it on the baking sheet. Repeat with the remaining onion slices.
6. Place the sheet in the preheated oven and bake for 6 minutes. Turn each slice over and bake for 4 minutes more, or until crispy.
7. Serve warm.

Serves 2. Prep time: 5 minutes. Cook time: 10 minutes

PER SERVING (½ FINISHED RECIPE): CALORIES: 210 / TOTAL FAT: 14.1G /
CARBOHYDRATES: 6.4G / FIBER: 3.2G / PROTEIN: 6.3G

VEGETABLE CHIPS

QUICK
& EASY

IMMUNITY
BOOST

THYROID
SUPPORT

KIDNEY
SUPPORT

These crunchy chips are more flavorful and nutritious than conventional potato chips. And, because they're baked, not fried, they fall perfectly within the guidelines of the Alkaline Diet. Serve them with Spinach-Artichoke Dip (page 102) or Healthy Hummus (page 103). Feel free to use other root vegetables and have fun experimenting.

Recipe Tip Toss these chips with garlic powder, chili powder, curry powder, or other alkaline-friendly seasonings to add variety.

1 parsnip, peeled

1 large carrot, peeled

1 beet, peeled

1 sweet potato, peeled

1 teaspoon sea salt

Cooking spray

1. Preheat the oven to 375°F.
2. Using a food processor attachment, mandoline, or food slicer, slice the parsnip, carrot, beet, and sweet potato into very thin slices. Lay the slices flat on a paper towel and sprinkle with the salt. Cover with more paper towel and let sit for 15 minutes.
3. Blot any moisture on the vegetable slices.
4. Spray a baking sheet with cooking spray.
5. Place the vegetable slices in a single layer on the baking sheet. Spray the vegetables with cooking spray.
6. Place the sheet in the preheated oven and bake for about 20 minutes, or until crisp.

Serves 4. Prep time: 5 minutes. Cook time: 20 minutes

PER SERVING (¼ OF FINISHED RECIPE): CALORIES: 69 / TOTAL FAT: 0.2G /
CARBOHYDRATES: 16.1G / FIBER: 3.5G / PROTEIN: 1.4G

SWEET POTATO FRIES

IMMUNITY
BOOST

THYROID
SUPPORT

KIDNEY
SUPPORT

Sweet potato fries are all the rage these days. It's no wonder, since one potato contains more than twice the daily requirement of vitamin A. These baked fries are so easy and delicious, you won't miss the fryer. For variation, sprinkle them with garlic powder, chili powder, nutritional yeast, or stevia mixed with cinnamon.

Recipe Tip There is a difference between sweet potatoes and yams. Sweet potatoes have an orange flesh and yams have a white flesh. Both are delicious when made into fries.

2 sweet potatoes, peeled and cut into fries

Cooking spray
1 teaspoon sea salt

1. Preheat the oven to 425°F.
2. Spray a baking sheet with cooking spray.
3. Place the fries in a single layer on the sheet. Coat the fries with cooking spray and sprinkle with the salt.
4. Place the sheet in the preheated oven and bake for 15 minutes. Turn the fries over. Cook for 15 minutes more, or until crisp. Serve.

Serves 2. Prep time: 10 minutes. Cook time: 30 minutes

PER SERVING (½ FINISHED RECIPE): CALORIES: 71 / TOTAL FAT: 0.02G / CARBOHYDRATES: 5.8G / FIBER: 0.3G / PROTEIN: 2.1G

SANTA'S GINGER SNAPS

QUICK
& EASY

IMMUNITY
BOOST

THYROID
SUPPORT

KIDNEY
SUPPORT

Bet you didn't think you could have cookies that were alkaline friendly! Well, the ingredients for these treats are all on the "Go" list. These ginger snaps are so tender and delicious that you won't want to share them with Santa. Serve with some chilled almond milk and feel like a kid again!

Recipe Tip Don't use fresh ginger in this recipe. It won't mix in as well with the ingredients and you'll be left with chunks of strong ginger in the cookie.

½ cup almond flour

⅓ cup coconut flour

⅓ cup coconut sugar

2 tablespoons arrowroot powder

½ teaspoon baking soda

½ teaspoon ground ginger

½ teaspoon cinnamon

¼ teaspoon sea salt

¼ teaspoon cloves

¼ cup coconut oil

3 tablespoons ground flaxseed, soaked in 3 tablespoons warm water

1. Preheat the oven to 350°F.
2. Line a baking sheet with parchment paper.
3. In a large bowl, mix together the almond flour, coconut flour, coconut sugar, arrowroot, baking soda, ginger, cinnamon, salt, and cloves.
4. In a microwaveable bowl, melt the coconut oil by microwaving on high for 30 seconds. Combine this with the flaxseed mixture. Add the coconut oil mixture to the bowl with the dry ingredients. Stir to combine. The dough will be stiff.
5. Scoop the dough by tablespoonfuls and roll by hand into balls. Place the dough balls onto the prepared baking sheet and flatten into discs.
6. Place the sheet into the preheated oven and bake for 10 to 15 minutes, or until firm.
7. Let cool before serving.

Serves 6. Prep time: 10 minutes. Cook time: 10 to 15 minutes

PER SERVING (2 COOKIES): CALORIES: 174 / TOTAL FAT: 10.4G / CARBOHYDRATES: 17.2G / FIBER: 1.7G / PROTEIN: 2.8G

SNICKERDOODLE COOKIES

QUICK
& EASY

IMMUNITY
BOOST

THYROID
SUPPORT

KIDNEY
SUPPORT

This recipe takes the basic cookie ingredients and adds yummy variations on the theme. Feel free to experiment by adding foods on the "Go" list. Here, the classic Snickerdoodle sugar cookie is reinvented with an intense vanilla flavor.

½ cup almond flour

⅓ cup coconut flour

⅔ cup coconut sugar, divided

2 tablespoons arrowroot powder

½ teaspoon baking soda

¼ teaspoon sea salt

1 teaspoon cinnamon

¼ cup coconut oil

3 tablespoons ground flaxseed, soaked in 3 tablespoons warm water

1 vanilla bean, split lengthwise and seeds scraped out

1. Preheat the oven to 350°F.
2. Line a baking sheet with parchment paper.
3. In a large bowl, mix together the almond flour, coconut flour, ⅓ cup coconut sugar, arrowroot, baking soda, and salt.
4. In a small bowl, add the remaining ⅓ cup coconut sugar and the cinnamon. Stir to combine. Set aside.
5. In a microwaveable bowl, melt the coconut oil by microwaving on high for 30 seconds. Add the flaxseed mixture and vanilla bean seeds. Stir to combine.
6. Stir the coconut oil mixture into the bowl with the dry ingredients. Mix to combine. The dough will be stiff.
7. Shape the dough by hand into 1-inch balls. Roll each dough ball into the reserved cinnamon sugar. Place them on the prepared baking sheet about 1½ inches apart.
8. Place the baking sheet in the preheated oven and bake for 10 to 12 minutes, or until the tops are browned.
9. Cool on a wire rack and serve.

Serves 6. Prep time: 10 minutes. Cook time: 10 to 12 minutes

PER SERVING (2 COOKIES): CALORIES: 174 / TOTAL FAT: 10.4G / CARBOHYDRATES: 17.2G / FIBER: 1.7G / PROTEIN: 2.8G

BETTER THAN GIRL SCOUT COOKIES

IMMUNITY
BOOST

THYROID
SUPPORT

KIDNEY
SUPPORT

This recipe is a little more complicated than some others in this book. The advantage of this recipe is that it's a raw recipe, meaning it's not baked. Because the recipe contains alkalized cocoa powder, these cookies count as part of your 20 percent. Freeze any leftovers to practice portion control on these delicious, healthy treats.

Recipe Tip Dutch-processing uses potassium carbonate to neutralize the high acidity of cocoa to a pH of 7. Look for Dutch-processed cocoa in your local market or under Resources.

For the cookie base

1 cup dried shredded unsweetened coconut

1 cup raw almonds

2 pinches sea salt

2½ tablespoons coconut oil, melted

1 packet stevia

For the coconut caramel layer

½ cup dried shredded unsweetened coconut

8 Medjool dates

1 tablespoon water, plus additional as needed

2 tablespoons coconut oil, melted

Pinch sea salt

For the chocolate icing

4 tablespoons coconut oil, melted

1 packet stevia

4 tablespoons unsweetened Dutch-processed cocoa powder

To make the cookie base:

1. Line a baking sheet with parchment paper.
2. In a food processor, blend the coconut for 60 seconds. Add the almonds and salt and blend until they are ground into a meal. Blend in the coconut oil and stevia until a dough forms.
3. Roll the dough between two sheets of wax paper to a ¼-inch thickness. Freeze the dough for 10 minutes, or until firm.
4. Using a round cookie cutter, cut out 12 cookies. Place each cookie base on the parchment-lined baking sheet.

continued →

To make the coconut caramel layer:

1. Preheat the oven to 350°F.
2. On another baking sheet, spread the coconut in an even layer. Toast it in the preheated oven for 5 minutes, taking care that it doesn't burn. Remove and cool.
3. In a food processor, add the dates, water, and coconut oil. Blend to combine. Add the salt and more water, if needed. Continue to blend until the mixture resembles caramel. Add the toasted coconut and mix to combine.
4. Spread an equal layer of the caramel-coconut mixture onto each cookie base.

To make the chocolate icing:

1. In a small bowl, mix together the coconut oil, stevia, and cocoa powder.
2. With a spoon, drizzle the icing over each of the 12 cookies.
3. Refrigerate the cookies for 10 minutes to solidify the layers before eating.

Serves 12. Prep time: 30 minutes. Cook time: 5 minutes, to toast the coconut

---

PER SERVING (1 COOKIE): CALORIES: 180 / TOTAL FAT: 16.9G / CARBOHYDRATES: 7.4G / FIBER: 2.3G / PROTEIN: 2.2G

BANANA MUFFINS

QUICK
& EASY

IMMUNITY
BOOST

THYROID
SUPPORT

KIDNEY
SUPPORT

These muffins are made with almond butter, which can be found near the peanut butter in most markets. Make sure you get a brand with no added sugar or oil. Also, use muffin liners sprayed with cooking spray so they come out of the pan more easily. Freeze any leftovers (if you have them!) for a quick, on-the-go healthy treat.

Recipe Tip When your bananas are starting to get ripe, peel them and freeze them. You can use them in smoothies or banana "ice cream," but you can also use them in this muffin recipe. They get a bit mushy, but since they're blended, it doesn't matter.

Cooking spray

2 ripe bananas

1 cup dates

½ cup roasted creamy almond butter

½ cup coconut flour

¼ cup coconut oil, melted

2 teaspoons baking soda

½ teaspoon sea salt

1 vanilla bean, split lengthwise and seeds scraped out

1. Preheat the oven to 350°F.
2. Line a muffin pan with paper liners and spray the liners with cooking spray.
3. In a food processor, add the bananas and dates and blend until smooth.
4. Add the almond butter, coconut flour, coconut oil, baking soda, salt, and vanilla bean seeds to the processor and pulse until a thick batter forms.
5. With an ice cream scoop, scoop the batter into the lined muffin tins, filling each two-thirds full.
6. Place the muffins in the preheated oven and bake for 15 to 18 minutes, or until a toothpick inserted into a muffin comes out clean.
7. Cool and serve.

Serves 12. Prep time: 5 minutes. Cook time: 15 to 18 minutes

PER SERVING (1 MUFFIN): CALORIES: 181 / TOTAL FAT: 10.1G / CARBOHYDRATES: 21.7.4G / FIBER: 2.6G / PROTEIN: 3.8G

ALMOND–QUINOA MUFFINS

QUICK
& EASY

IMMUNITY
BOOST

THYROID
SUPPORT

KIDNEY
SUPPORT

The quinoa adds a slight crunch to these muffins that is reminiscent of a poppy seed muffin. It also adds a ton of protein to keep you going all morning long. This isn't a very sweet muffin and is a great alternative when you don't want something overly sweet but don't want something savory either. As with the other muffin recipe, use sprayed liners so that the muffins come out without sticking.

Recipe Tip If you prefer your muffins a little bit sweeter, add a packet of stevia to the batter and mix well.

Cooking spray

1 cup vanilla almond milk

¼ cup applesauce

1 tablespoon ground flaxseed

1 vanilla bean, split lengthwise and seeds
 scraped out

1¼ cups coconut flour

¼ cup almond flour

1½ teaspoons baking powder

½ teaspoon sea salt

½ teaspoon ground cinnamon

1¼ cups cooked quinoa

1. Preheat the oven to 350°F.
2. Line a muffin pan with paper liners and spray the liners with cooking spray.
3. In a food processor, place the almond milk, applesauce, flaxseed, and vanilla bean seeds. Blend until smooth.
4. In a medium bowl, mix together the coconut flour, almond flour, baking powder, salt, and cinnamon. Add these dry ingredients to the food processor and pulse until a batter forms.
5. Add the quinoa and mix until blended completely.
6. With an ice cream scoop, scoop the batter into the lined muffin pan, filling each two-thirds full.
7. Place the pan in the preheated oven and bake for 15 to 18 minutes, or until a toothpick inserted comes out clean.
8. Cool and serve.

Serves 12. Prep time: 15 minutes. Cook time: 15 to 18 minutes

PER SERVING (1 MUFFIN): CALORIES: 170 / TOTAL FAT: 6.1G / CARBOHYDRATES: 24.9G / FIBER: 2.3G / PROTEIN: 4.5G

SELF-FROSTING CARROT CAKE

IMMUNITY
BOOST

THYROID
SUPPORT

KIDNEY
SUPPORT

This cake is amazingly moist because of the water content of the pineapple and carrots. The secret is to make the cake batter first and then add the pineapple to the center so the juice is evenly mixed. This cake self-frosts by forming a topping that is made when you turn the cake upside down. With this recipe, you can have your cake and be healthy eating it too!

Recipe Tip If you don't have crushed pineapple on hand, you can use canned pineapple chunks or even rings by processing them in a food processor.

Cooking spray

⅓ cup coconut oil plus 3 tablespoons, melted, divided

½ cup grated carrot

1¼ cups almond flour

1½ teaspoons baking powder

¼ teaspoon sea salt

1 (8-ounce) can crushed pineapple in juice, drained, juice reserved (about ¾ cup)

½ cup flaked unsweetened coconut

⅓ cup chopped almonds

1. Preheat the oven to 350°F.
2. Spray an 8-inch round cake pan with cooking spray.
3. In a large bowl, combine ⅓ cup coconut oil and the carrot.
4. In a medium bowl, sift together the almond flour, baking powder, and salt. Add these dry ingredients to the carrot-oil mixture, then add the reserved pineapple juice. Mix well after each addition.
5. Spread half of batter in the prepared pan. Add the crushed pineapple in an even layer over the batter. Top with the remaining cake batter.
6. In a small bowl, combine the coconut, almonds, and the remaining 3 tablespoons coconut oil. Sprinkle the almond mixture evenly over the cake.

continued →

Self-Frosting Carrot Cake *continued*

7. Place the pan in the preheated oven and bake for 35 to 40 minutes, or until a cake tester comes out clean.
8. Carefully flip the pan upside down onto a cake plate to reveal a perfectly cake!

Serves 8. Prep time: 15 minutes. Cook time: 35 to 40 minutes

PER SERVING (⅛ OF FINISHED CAKE): CALORIES: 282 / TOTAL FAT: 26.6G /
CARBOHYDRATES: 10.3G / FIBER: 3.2G / PROTEIN: 4.8G

PUMPKIN–RHUBARB PIE

IMMUNITY
BOOST

THYROID
SUPPORT

KIDNEY
SUPPORT

This is not a sweet pie, but is instead savory. In many parts of the world, pumpkin is eaten like any other gourd or squash. The addition of rhubarb adds a nice tartness, as well as making the pie a beautiful color. Use the All-Purpose Pie Crust (page 181) as a base. You can also serve this crustless.

Recipe Tip For an exotic presentation, bake this pie inside a scooped out pumpkin, omitting the crust.

1 All-Purpose Pie Crust (page 181)

1 bunch rhubarb, trimmed and chopped

1 (8-ounce) can pumpkin purée

1 teaspoon nutmeg

1 teaspoon cinnamon

1 teaspoon ginger

1 teaspoon chili powder

1 teaspoon freshly ground black pepper

Dash sea salt

1 packet stevia

1. Preheat the oven to 350°F.
2. Line an 8-inch pie plate with the prepared crust.
3. Bring a medium pot filled with water to a boil. When the water boils, remove the pot from heat, add the rhubarb to the water, and let sit for 4 minutes. Drain the rhubarb.
4. In a food processor, place the rhubarb, pumpkin, nutmeg, cinnamon, ginger, chili powder, pepper, salt, and stevia. Blend until smooth.
5. Pour the mixture over the pie crust. Cover with aluminum foil.
6. Place the pan in the preheated oven and bake for 30 minutes.
7. Cool completely, and serve.

Serves 8. Prep time: 10 minutes. Cook time: 30 minutes

PER SERVING (⅛ OF FINISHED PIE WITH CRUST): CALORIES: 148 / TOTAL FAT: 9.8G /
CARBOHYDRATES: 38G / FIBER: 6.9G / PROTEIN: 11.6G

BAKED APPLES AND RAISINS

QUICK
& EASY

IMMUNITY
BOOST

THYROID
SUPPORT

KIDNEY
SUPPORT

They say an apple a day keeps the doctor away. With this baked dish, you'll find yourself hanging out in Hotel Delicious instead of a hospital. These apples are also great cold, topped with some Coconut Whipped Cream (page 202). You can use any kind of apple you wish, but Granny Smith tends to hold up best when baking.

Recipe Tip There are two kinds of raisins, brown and golden. Brown raisins come from red grapes and golden ones come from green grapes. Use both for an extra serving of micronutrients.

2 apples, tops removed and reserved

¼ cup raisins

1 teaspoon cinnamon

1 packet stevia

1. Preheat the oven to 350°F.
2. With a spoon, scoop out the insides of the apples and place the contents into a medium bowl, discarding the core and seeds. Be careful to leave enough apple inside the skin so you have a shell and the skin is not pierced.
3. In the medium bowl, add the raisins, cinnamon, and stevia and mix together with the scooped-out apple pieces.
4. Spoon the apple mixture, evenly divided, back into the apple shells. Cover each with a reserved top.
5. Place the apples in a baking pan and bake for 15 minutes, or until the apples are soft.
6. Cool slightly and serve warm.

Serves 2. Prep time: 5 minutes. Cook time: 15 minutes

PER SERVING (1 FILLED APPLE): CALORIES: 95 / CARBOHYDRATES: 25.1G / FIBER: 4.4G

ROASTED GARLIC CABBAGE

IMMUNITY
BOOST

THYROID
SUPPORT

KIDNEY
SUPPORT

This dish is so easy and delicious you'll wonder why you never thought of it before. Simply slice a head of cabbage, season it, and bake it. If you're not a fan of cabbage, definitely try this recipe and see if it changes your mind. You can serve this as a plate underneath the Curried Eggplant (page 165) or roasted vegetables.

Recipe Tip Try using purple cabbage instead of green; it basically tastes the same but offers a more dramatic presentation.

1 (2-pound) head organic green cabbage, cut into 1-inch-thick slices (about 8 slices)

1½ tablespoons coconut oil

2 to 3 large garlic cloves, smashed

Pinch sea salt

1. Preheat the oven to 425°F.
2. Place the cabbage slices in a baking pan and brush on both sides with the coconut oil.
3. Rub each cabbage slice with garlic and sprinkle with salt.
4. Place the pan in the preheated oven and roast for 20 minutes. Flip the cabbage slices over. Roast for another 20 to 25 minutes, until the edges are brown and crisp.

Serves 4. Prep time: 5 minutes. Cook time: 45 minutes

PER SERVING (2 CABBAGE SLICES): CALORIES: 90 / TOTAL FAT: 5.3G /
CARBOHYDRATES: 10.3G / FIBER: 4.5G / PROTEIN: 2.3G

QUICK
& EASY

IMMUNITY
BOOST

KIDNEY
SUPPORT

CINCO DE MAYO CASSEROLE

This is a great recipe to bring to a party when you're not sure there will be alkaline-friendly food for you to eat. The quinoa is mixed with traditional Mexican ingredients for an authentic flair. And, since there is no cheese or sour cream, it fits perfectly with your eating plan.

Recipe Tip If you didn't sprout your beans, don't worry. You can use regular, canned black beans. Just consider this recipe part of your 20 percent if you use canned beans.

2 cups cooked quinoa

¼ cup sprouted black beans (see page 201)

¼ cup chopped fresh cilantro

½ red onion, chopped

½ teaspoon ground cumin

1 avocado, mashed

½ teaspoon sea salt

Juice of 1 lime

1 cup Salsa Fresca (page 198)

Assorted raw vegetables, for serving

1. In a medium bowl, combine the quinoa, beans, cilantro, red onion, and cumin.
2. In a small bowl, combine the avocado, salt, and lime juice.
3. Spread the quinoa mixture into the bottom of a serving dish. Top with the avocado and salsa.
4. Serve accompanied by the raw vegetables.

Serves 6. Prep time: 15 minutes

PER SERVING (½ CUP): CALORIES: 309 / TOTAL FAT: 10.8G / CARBOHYDRATES: 45.8G / FIBER: 8.1G / PROTEIN: 10.7G

THE MONSTER MASH

This is the ultimate comfort food. The recipe contains warming layers of mashed vegetables. Curl up by a fire with a plate of this and some warm tea and let the vitamins and minerals heal you from the inside. Freeze any leftovers so you can have this on hand after a tough day.

Recipe Tip Add a layer of mashed baby or new potatoes if you wish. If you add these new foods, you'll just need to update the recipe's nutritional information.

1 sweet potato, peeled and diced

2 cups cooked cauliflower florets

1 cup almond milk, room temperature, divided, plus additional as needed

1 teaspoon sea salt, divided

2 cups cooked broccoli florets

1. Place the sweet potato in a small pan of water. Bring the water to a boil. Cook the sweet potato for 7 minutes, or until it is soft. Drain and set aside.
2. While the sweet potato is cooking, place the cauliflower in a large mixing bowl. Add ⅓ cup almond milk and ⅓ teaspoon salt. Mash the cauliflower until smooth, adding additional almond milk if needed. Remove from the mixing bowl and set aside.
3. In the same large mixing bowl, add the broccoli, ⅓ cup almond milk, and ⅓ teaspoon salt. Mash the broccoli until smooth. Remove from the mixing bowl and set aside.
4. In the same large mixing bowl, add the warm sweet potatoes, the remaining ⅓ cup almond milk, and the remaining ⅓ teaspoon salt. Mash the sweet potato until smooth.
5. Place one-half of the mashed sweet potato in the bottom of each of two medium bowls. Add one-half of the mashed cauliflower to each bowl on top of the sweet potato. Layer that with one-half of the mashed broccoli in each bowl. Serve warm.

Serves 2. Prep time: 15 minutes. Cook time: 7 minutes

PER SERVING (½ FINISHED RECIPE): CALORIES: 158 / TOTAL FAT: 0.5G /
CARBOHYDRATES: 27.1G / FIBER 6.8G / PROTEIN: 7.7G

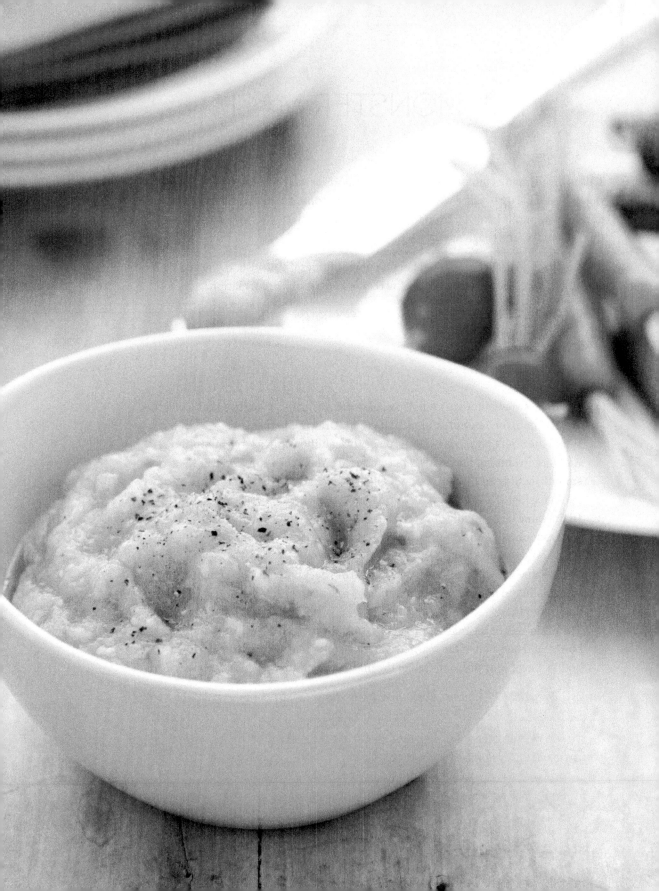

6

DIY SNACKS

SUSHI HAND ROLL

QUICK
& EASY

IMMUNITY
BOOST

THYROID
SUPPORT

KIDNEY
SUPPORT

Traditional sushi rice is usually white rice, seasoned with a sweet vinegar. Since those foods are on the "No Go" list, brown rice is substituted here. Soy sauce is also an acid-producing food, so this recipe calls for sesame oil and sesame seeds. Wasabi is a spicy condiment that is alkaline-producing. Use it sparingly as it is intense.

Recipe Tip You can use quinoa instead of the brown rice for a change of pace.

2 nori seaweed squares

¼ cup cooked brown rice, divided

Wasabi, for garnish (optional)

½ avocado, diced, divided

½ cucumber, peeled and diced, divided

1 teaspoon sesame oil, divided

1 teaspoon toasted sesame seeds, divided

1. Place one nori sheet in your hand. Add 2 tablespoons brown rice, wasabi (if using), half of the diced avocado, and half of the diced cucumber.
2. Drizzle with ½ teaspoon of sesame oil. Sprinkle ½ teaspoon of the sesame seeds.
3. Wrap the nori around the filling so it looks like a cone. Carefully set on a plate.
4. Repeat with the remaining ingredients for a second hand roll.
5. Serve and eat immediately.

Serves 1. Prep time: 10 minutes

PER SERVING: CALORIES: 457 / TOTAL FAT: 27.1G / CARBOHYDRATES: 51.1G / FIBER: 9.5G / PROTEIN: 7G

PARTY MIX

QUICK
& EASY

IMMUNITY
BOOST

THYROID
SUPPORT

KIDNEY
SUPPORT

The whole point of a party is to have fun. But who can have fun feeling guilty about eating acid-producing unhealthy food? Instead, serve or bring this party mix and celebrate healthy living with your friends. It's filled with fiber, vitamins, minerals, and protein. But, mostly, it's filled with party fun.

Recipe Tip You can get dried, roasted peas in the Asian food section of your local market. Try the wasabi flavored ones to make it spicy!

Cooking spray

1 cup raw almonds

½ cup flaked unsweetened coconut

1 cup raisins

1 cup dried pineapple pieces

½ cup roasted peas

½ cup pumpkin seeds

2 tablespoons garlic powder

2 tablespoons onion powder

1 teaspoon chili powder

1 teaspoon ground ginger

1 teaspoon sea salt

1 tablespoon coconut oil

1. Preheat the oven to 425°F.
2. Spray a large baking pan with cooking spray.
3. In a medium bowl, combine the almonds, coconut, raisins, pineapple, peas, pumpkin seeds, garlic powder, onion powder, chili powder, ginger, salt, and coconut oil.
4. Spread the mix in an even layer in the baking pan.
5. Bake for 10 minutes in the preheated oven, being careful that it doesn't burn.
6. Remove from the oven and cool before serving.

Serves 6. Prep time: 5 minutes. Cook time: 10 minutes

PER SERVING (¾ CUP): CALORIES: 227 / TOTAL FAT: 12.7G / CARBOHYDRATES: 27.9G / FIBER: 4.1G / PROTEIN: 5.1G

HERBED CRACKERS

IMMUNITY
BOOST

THYROID
SUPPORT

KIDNEY
SUPPORT

It's so easy to make your own crackers that you won't even miss the stale-tasting ones that come out of a box. These pack a nutritional fiber-filled punch. The rosemary is said to lower blood pressure. The flaxseed is a great source of fatty acids, which are necessary for the body's health. Serve with Spinach-Artichoke Dip (page 102) or Healthy Hummus (page 103).

Recipe Tip If you don't have flaxseed meal, grind flaxseeds in a clean coffee grinder or small food processor. When mixed with water, flaxseed acts as a thickener.

2 tablespoons flaxseed meal

4 tablespoons water

1 tablespoon coconut oil

1 cup almond flour

1½ teaspoons fresh rosemary

¾ teaspoon finely chopped fresh oregano

¾ teaspoon finely chopped fresh thyme

1 tablespoon sesame seeds (optional)

½ teaspoon sea salt

1. Preheat the oven to 325°F.
2. In a small bowl, combine the flaxseed meal, water, and coconut oil. Refrigerate for 10 minutes until the mixture thickens.
3. In a medium bowl, combine the almond flour, rosemary, oregano, thyme, and sesame seeds (if using). Stir in the flaxseed mixture, combining thoroughly.
4. Shape the dough into a ball. On parchment paper, roll the dough to a ⅛-inch thickness. Sprinkle with the salt.
5. Place the parchment with the dough on a baking sheet. Cut the dough into 24 crackers of equal size, being careful not to cut through the parchment.
6. Place the baking sheet in the preheated oven. Bake for 20 minutes, watching closely to make sure the crackers don't burn.
7. Remove from the oven and cool.

Serves 6. Prep time: 15 minutes. Cook time: 20 minutes

PER SERVING (4 CRACKERS): CALORIES: 118 / TOTAL FAT: 4G / CARBOHYDRATES: 17.3G / FIBER: 1.6G / PROTEIN: 2.9G

SPINACH–ARTICHOKE DIP

QUICK
& EASY

IMMUNITY
BOOST

KIDNEY
SUPPORT

This party and restaurant staple typically is made with fat-laden, acid-producing cheese. It's usually so salty that all you taste is fat and salt—where are the veggies? This version tastes creamy (without any dairy!), and you can actually taste the delicious spinach and artichoke flavors. Packed with nutrition and taste, you may never eat the other version again. Just be sure to leave off the tomatoes if you're following the Thyroid-Support Plan.

Recipe Tip You can use frozen spinach in this recipe if you prefer. Just be sure to squeeze out all of the water.

Cooking spray

¾ cup raw cashews

¾ cup unsweetened almond milk

2 tablespoons freshly squeezed
  lemon juice

1 garlic clove

¾ teaspoon sea salt

1 tablespoon nutritional yeast

2 cups artichoke hearts, frozen or
  canned in water, not oil

2 cups baby spinach leaves

1 cup baby tomatoes

1. Preheat the oven to 425°F.
2. Spray a medium baking dish with cooking spray.
3. In a blender, combine the cashews, almond milk, lemon juice, garlic, salt, and yeast. Blend until very smooth.
4. Add the artichoke hearts, spinach, and tomatoes to the blender. Pulse to combine, but still leaving chunks of vegetables.
5. Transfer the dip to the prepared baking dish. Place the dish in the preheated oven and bake for 20 minutes.
6. Remove from the oven, cool for 5 minutes, and serve warm.

Serves 6. Prep time: 10 minutes. Cook time: 20 minutes

PER SERVING (¼ CUP): CALORIES: 178 / TOTAL FAT: 15.3G / CARBOHYDRATES: 10.3G / FIBER: 2.3G / PROTEIN: 4.4G

HEALTHY HUMMUS

QUICK
& EASY

IMMUNITY
BOOST

KIDNEY
SUPPORT

Traditional hummus is pretty healthy already. But, since chickpeas are one of those foods you should limit, this version adds some eggplant to boost the flavor while limiting the beans. Doing so makes this recipe taste like a delicious combination of hummus and baba ganoush. To roast the eggplant, put it in on a baking sheet, and bake in a 350°F oven for 30 minutes, or until it's soft.

Recipe Tip If you're on the Thyroid-Support Plan, omit the eggplant and substitute an extra cup of chickpeas instead.

1 cup chickpeas, canned or cooked

1 cup eggplant, roasted and peeled

1 garlic clove

1 tablespoon sesame oil

1 tablespoon freshly squeezed lemon juice

1 teaspoon sea salt

Water, for thinning

In a food processor, combine the chickpeas, eggplant, garlic, sesame oil, lemon juice, and salt. Blend until creamy smooth. Add water, if needed, to create a creamy consistency.

Serves 4. Prep time: 5 minutes

PER SERVING (½ CUP): CALORIES: 219 / TOTAL FAT: 6.5G / CARBOHYDRATES: 31.9G / FIBER: 9.5G / PROTEIN: 9.9G

QUICK
& EASY

IMMUNITY
BOOST

THYROID
SUPPORT

KIDNEY
SUPPORT

TEA PARTY CUCUMBER SANDWICHES

Aren't tea parties fun? Unfortunately, afternoon tea is usually an excuse to eat sugary, high-fat foods. Instead, serve these breadless sandwiches with tea, and perhaps some of the cookies from this book. You can indulge in a relaxing afternoon and be happy knowing you're supporting your health.

Recipe Tip You can quickly cook the asparagus in the microwave and then run it under cold water to cool it.

½ cup Healthy Hummus (page 103)
1 cucumber, peeled and sliced into
  ¼-inch rounds

4 asparagus spears, trimmed, cooked,
  cooled, and finely chopped

1. Place 1 teaspoon of hummus atop one cucumber round. Top with ½ teaspoon of the asparagus. Place a second cucumber round on top. Carefully place the sandwich on a serving plate.
2. Repeat with the remaining ingredients.

Serves 2. Prep time: 10 minutes

PER SERVING (4 SANDWICHES): CALORIES: 126 / TOTAL FAT: 6.2G / CARBOHYDRATES: 14.4G / FIBER: 4.5G / PROTEIN: 5.9G

MANGO–BARBECUE SLIDERS

One of the things many people miss when following the Alkaline Diet is meat. While this recipe doesn't contain any meat, it definitely provides that hearty barbecue flavor that is so satisfying. Bring this dish to a cookout and listen to everyone say, "That looks great!" These are very messy, so have lots of napkins on hand.

Recipe Tip If you don't have zucchini, substitute 1 cup of cooked, shredded spaghetti squash instead.

1 mango, peeled, pitted, and cut into large pieces

¼ cup Homemade Barbecue Sauce (page 207)

1 zucchini, peeled and julienned

4 portobello mushroom caps, gills removed

1. Preheat a grill or a grill pan on the stovetop to medium heat.
2. In a food processor, purée the mango. Add the Homemade Barbecue Sauce. Transfer the mixture to a medium bowl. Add the zucchini and mix well to combine.
3. Fill 1 mushroom cap with half of the mango-zucchini mixture. Top with another mushroom cap.
4. Repeat with remaining ingredients for a second slider.
5. Place the sliders on the grill and cook for 10 minutes, or until the desired level of tenderness.
6. Serve and eat immediately.

Serves 2. Prep time: 5 minutes. Cook time: 10 minutes

PER SERVING (1 SLIDER): CALORIES: 135 / TOTAL FAT: 0.6G / CARBOHYDRATES: 32.2G / FIBER: 3.1G / PROTEIN: 1.7G

QUICK
& EASY

IMMUNITY
BOOST

THYROID
SUPPORT

KIDNEY
SUPPORT

MOVIE NIGHT CAULIFLOWER POPCORN

There are few things more fun than settling in with a good movie and a bowl of popcorn. But, since corn is on the "No Go" list, what can you do? Try this recipe that uses roasted cauliflower instead of popcorn. Top it with garlic powder, chili powder, or nutritional yeast.

Recipe Tip Don't use frozen cauliflower for this recipe. It will be too soggy.

1 cauliflower head, separated into small florets

3 tablespoons coconut oil
1 teaspoon sea salt

1. Preheat the oven to 400°F.
2. In a large bowl, combine the cauliflower, coconut oil, and salt.
3. Transfer the cauliflower to a baking sheet and spread it evenly into a single layer.
4. Place the sheet in the preheated oven and roast for about 30 minutes, until golden brown and slightly crisp.

Serves 4. Prep time: 10 minutes. Cook time: 30 minutes

PER SERVING (ABOUT 1 CUP): CALORIES: 107 / TOTAL FAT: 10.3G / CARBOHYDRATES: 3.5G / FIBER: 1.7G / PROTEIN: 1.3G

BANANA CANDY COINS

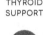

Sometimes you just want something sweet and you want it now. With these delectable treats, you don't have to wait to bake a cake or a batch of cookies. You can be eating a sweet treat that will help your health in 5 minutes! For this recipe, choose bananas that are on the firm side.

Recipe Tip Try this recipe with plantains, the less sweet cousin of the banana. The coins will be slightly firmer and less sweet than those made with bananas.

2 tablespoons shredded
  unsweetened coconut

Pinch sea salt

2 tablespoons coconut oil

1 banana, peeled and sliced into
  ¼-inch-thick slices

1. On a plate, combine the coconut and salt.
2. In a medium pan set over medium heat, melt the coconut oil.
3. Press each banana slice into the coconut mixture until coated.
4. Gently place each slice into the heated coconut oil. Sauté for 2 minutes, flip, and continue cooking for 2 to 3 minutes on the second side.
5. Cool slightly and serve warm.

Serves 1. Prep time: 2 minutes. Cook time: 5 minutes

PER SERVING: CALORIES: 171 / TOTAL FAT: 6.3G / CARBOHYDRATES: 28.4G / FIBER: 4.4G / PROTEIN: 1.5G

CHILE—LIME MANGO SLAW

QUICK
& EASY

IMMUNITY
BOOST

THYROID
SUPPORT

KIDNEY
SUPPORT

This dish is a twist on popular street food in Los Angeles and Mexico. Lime juice and a kick of chile powder liven up the sweet, crisp mango. If jicama is unfamiliar, get ready for a treat. This mild, crunchy root is great as a snack or in salads.

Recipe Tip If you're feeling lazy, skip the skewers and add the lime juice and chili powder straight onto mango that has been pitted and scored.

1 mango, peeled and cut into
  bite-size pieces
1 cup sliced jicama

1 cup sliced bell pepper
Juice of 1 lime
1 tablespoon chili powder

1. In a small bowl, combine mango, bell pepper, and jicama.
2. Squeeze the lime juice over the vegetables. Sprinkle with the chili powder.
3. Refrigerate for 15 minutes to allow flavors to blend and enjoy.

Serves 1. Prep time: 5 minutes. Cooling time: 15 minutes

PER SERVING: CALORIES: 201 / TOTAL FAT: 1.3G / CARBOHYDRATES: 50G /
FIBER: 5G / PROTEIN: 2.8G

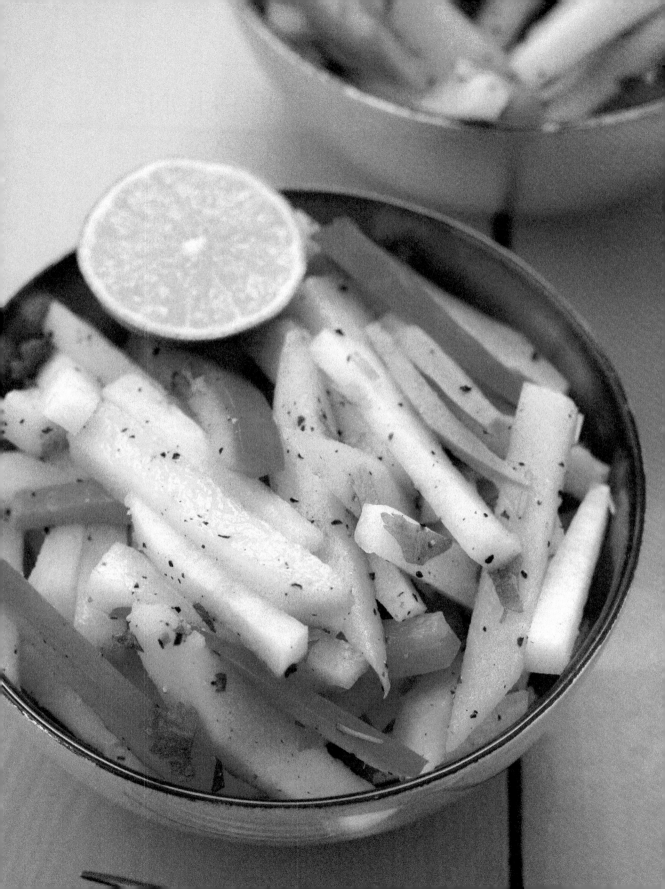

QUICK
& EASY

IMMUNITY
BOOST

KIDNEY
SUPPORT

HANG UP THE PHONE MINI-PIZZAS

There's no need to order in a pizza when you can have these delicious snacks. While they aren't a true replica of pizza because they don't have cheese, they will surely satisfy your craving in a way that is healthy. The tomato paste gives a healthy boost of lycopene, which is a powerful antioxidant. The mushroom caps act like a little bowl to hold all the delicious goodness.

Recipe Tip If you don't have tomato paste, you can substitute jarred pizza sauce. Just be sure to use a brand with no added oil or sugar.

Cooking spray

1 (6-ounce) can organic tomato paste

1 tablespoon garlic powder

1 tablespoon onion powder

1 teaspoon dried oregano

4 tablespoons sun-dried tomatoes

½ teaspoon sea salt, plus a pinch, divided

4 portobello mushroom caps, gills removed

4 slices fresh tomato

1. Preheat the oven to 350°F.
2. Spray a baking pan with cooking spray.
3. In a small bowl, mix together the tomato paste, garlic powder, onion powder, oregano, sun-dried tomatoes, and sea salt.
4. Evenly divide the tomato mixture into the four mushroom caps. Top each with 1 tomato slice and a pinch of the sea salt.
5. Transfer the pizzas to the baking pan, place the pan in the preheated oven, and bake for 15 minutes, or until the pizzas are hot and bubbly.

Serves 4. Prep time: 5 minutes. Cook time: 15 minutes

PER SERVING (1 MINI-PIZZA): CALORIES: 66 / TOTAL FAT: 1.3G / CARBOHYDRATES: 13.4G / FIBER: 2.8G / PROTEIN: 2.9G

BUFFALO FLOWERS

IMMUNITY
BOOST

THYROID
SUPPORT

KIDNEY
SUPPORT

This is another one of those game-day staples. This alkaline-friendly version of Buffalo wings gives you the crunchy spice, without the acid-producing animal products. You can adjust the spiciness, if you wish, by reducing the amount of cayenne pepper. Serve with celery sticks and Ranch Dressing (page 211).

Recipe Tip Instead of the cayenne pepper, try your favorite brand of hot sauce. Just be sure to avoid traditional hot wing sauce as it's usually loaded with sugar and oil.

1 teaspoon sea salt

1 teaspoon garlic powder

1 teaspoon onion powder

1 cauliflower head, broken into florets

2 tablespoons coconut oil, melted

½ teaspoon cayenne pepper

1. Preheat the oven to 450°F.
2. In a small bowl, mix together the salt, garlic powder, and onion powder.
3. Season the cauliflower with the spice mix. Place the seasoned cauliflower in a baking pan and into the preheated oven. Bake for 10 minutes, turn the cauliflower over, and bake for 10 minutes more.
4. In a large bowl, while the cauliflower is baking, combine the coconut oil and cayenne pepper.
5. Transfer the hot cauliflower to the large bowl with the coconut oil. Toss to coat thoroughly and return the cauliflower to the baking pan.
6. Bake for 5 minutes more, until the sauce is absorbed.
7. Remove from the oven and let sit for 10 minutes before serving.

Serves 4. Prep time: 10 minutes. Cook time: 25 minutes

PER SERVING (ABOUT 1 CUP): CALORIES: 82 / TOTAL FAT: 6.9G / CARBOHYDRATES: 4.6G / FIBER: 1.8G / PROTEIN: 1.5G

QUICK
& EASY

IMMUNITY
BOOST

THYROID
SUPPORT

KIDNEY
SUPPORT

SZECHUAN GREEN BEANS

This classic Chinese restaurant staple makes a fantastic snack. This recipe puts a lighter twist on the original by roasting the beans instead of frying them. Healthy eating doesn't have to be boring, and these addictive beans are proof. Use fresh green beans rather than canned, so they aren't mushy.

Recipe Tip Try Chinese green beans for a change. They are found in the produce section of some markets.

1 pound green beans, ends trimmed

1 teaspoon coconut oil

1 teaspoon sesame oil

½ teaspoon red pepper flakes

2 garlic cloves, finely chopped

1 teaspoon chopped fresh ginger

½ teaspoon sea salt

1. Adjust the oven racks so that the top rack is closest to the broiler.
2. Preheat the broiler.
3. Place the green beans in a baking pan in a single layer. Broil the beans for about 10 minutes, or until they start to show black flecks. Remove the beans from the broiler and transfer them to a large bowl. Set aside.
4. In a small saucepan, add the coconut oil, sesame oil, red pepper flakes, garlic, ginger, and salt. Warm the mixture over medium heat until it begins to shimmer and turn red. Turn off the heat.
5. Pour the warm sauce over the green beans and toss well to combine.
6. Return the beans to the baking pan and place back under the broiler for 5 minutes.
7. Remove from the oven, place the green beans on a serving platter, and serve warm.

Serves 4. Prep time: 5 minutes. Cook time: 15 minutes

PER SERVING (4 OUNCES SAUCED GREEN BEANS): CALORIES: 60 / TOTAL FAT: 2.5G / CARBOHYDRATES: 9G / FIBER: 4G / PROTEIN: 2.2G

EGGPLANT ROLLUPS

These rollups make for a great afternoon snack or even a light lunch. These are served with a tapenade, which is usually made with olives. Since olives are on the "No Go" list, they are omitted here. The filling is high in vitamin C and is so good you might find yourself putting it on all kinds of other foods.

Recipe Tip To make sure you always have roasted red peppers on hand, just pop some in the oven in a baking pan and let them roast as you put away the other groceries. It should take about 15 minutes at 350°F.

For the tapenade
1 (12-ounce) jar packed-in-water roasted
  red peppers
¼ onion, chopped
1 garlic clove
1 tablespoon freshly squeezed lemon juice
¼ teaspoon red pepper flakes
3 fresh basil leaves

For the eggplant
2 eggplants, tops removed, thinly sliced
  lengthwise (about 24 slices)
Cooking spray
2 teaspoons sea salt

To make the tapenade:
In a food processor, add the roasted red peppers, onion, garlic, lemon juice, red pepper flakes, and basil. Pulse until blended but still chunky.

To make the eggplant:
1. Preheat the grill to medium, or preheat the broiler.
2. Lay the eggplant slices on a baking sheet and spray with cooking spray. Sprinkle with the salt.
3. Transfer the eggplant slices to the grill and grill for 3 minutes, or until grill marks form. If you don't have a grill, place the baking sheet in the broiler and broil instead.
4. Remove the eggplant from the grill and transfer it back to the baking sheet (or remove the baking sheet from the oven).

continued →

Eggplant Rollups *continued*

5. If using a grill, preheat the oven to 375°F.
6. If using a broiler for the eggplant slices, reduce the oven heat to 375°F.
7. Place 1 to 2 tablespoons of tapenade on one end of each eggplant slice. Roll the slices up and over the filling, finishing seam-side down. Put the sheet back in the oven and bake the rolls for 10 minutes or until heated.
8. Serve warm.

Serves 6. Prep time: 15 minutes. Cook time: 13 minutes

PER SERVING (4 ROLLS): CALORIES: 37 / TOTAL FAT: 0.3G / CARBOHYDRATES: 8.7G / FIBER: 3.5G / PROTEIN: 1.4G

MUSHROOM PÂTÉ

QUICK
& EASY

IMMUNITY
BOOST

THYROID
SUPPORT

KIDNEY
SUPPORT

Mushrooms are such a versatile food! They add a meaty flavor to most dishes. They're also a nutritional powerhouse, as they are loaded with essential nutrients such as vitamin D. Spread this pâté on Herbed Crackers (page 101) or Vegetable Chips (page 81).

Recipe Tip For variation, experiment with different kinds of mushrooms. Also, if you're feeling luxurious, drizzle a tiny bit of truffle oil on top before serving.

Cooking spray

1 onion, chopped

2 pounds fresh mushrooms, any kind, finely chopped

2 garlic cloves, minced

1 tablespoon chopped fresh parsley

¼ teaspoon finely chopped fresh rosemary

½ teaspoon sea salt

1 tablespoon freshly squeezed lemon juice

1. Spray a medium saucepan with the cooking spray. Add the onion and cook over medium heat for about 5 minutes, or until translucent.
2. Add the mushrooms and garlic to the pan. Cook for 10 minutes more, until cooked through.
3. Remove from the heat and transfer the mixture to a food processor. Add the parsley, rosemary, salt, and lemon juice. Pulse to a desired consistency.
4. Serve as suggested above.

Serves 6. Prep time: 5 minutes. Cook time: 15 minutes

PER SERVING (¼ CUP): CALORIES: 43 / TOTAL FAT: 0.6G / CARBOHYDRATES: 7.1G / FIBER 3.5G / PROTEIN: 5G

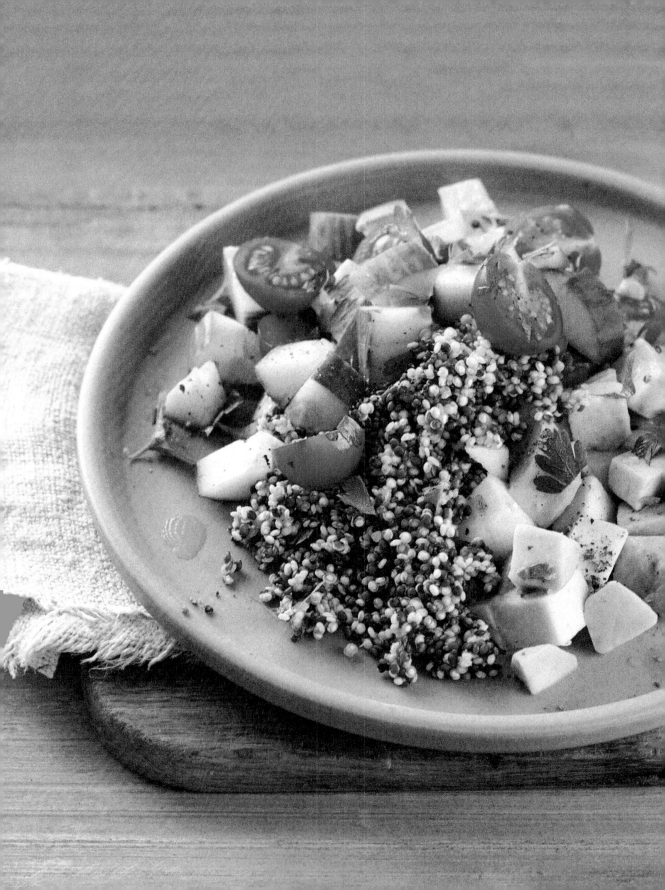

7

MEAL-SIZE SALADS

SALAD IN YOUR HAND

These perfectly portable lettuce wraps are great for when you don't want to hassle with utensils. Just pack everything together and assemble at the last minute. Feel free to substitute ingredients depending on what you have on "hand," remembering to skip the tomato if you're following the Thyroid-Support Plan. Serve with your favorite dressing from chapter 11 (see page 195).

Recipe Tip Let the lettuce come to room temperature before filling to make it easier to fold.

4 leaves lettuce, iceberg or Romaine

½ avocado, diced

1 carrot, peeled and shredded

½ tomato, diced

⅓ cucumber, peeled and diced

1 tablespoon chopped almonds

1. Lay the lettuce leaves out on a plate.
2. Fill each leaf with one-quarter each of the avocado, carrot, tomato, cucumber, and almonds. Wrap each leaf around its filling.
3. Eat and enjoy.

Serves 1. Prep time: 10 minutes

PER SERVING: CALORIES: 189 / TOTAL FAT: 13.1G / CARBOHYDRATES: 17.8G / FIBER: 6.5G / PROTEIN: 4.1G

SALAD ON A STICK

QUICK
& EASY

IMMUNITY
BOOST

KIDNEY
SUPPORT

You can serve this dish cold or warm. If you wish to grill these salad sticks, be sure to soak the skewers for 15 minutes prior to use so they don't burn on the grill. As with the other salad recipes in this chapter, feel free to substitute your favorite vegetables for the ones recommended here, but remember to omit the cherry tomatoes in all cases if you're following the Thyroid-Support Plan. Serve with your favorite dressing from chapter 11 (page 195).

Recipe Tip To make this recipe thyroid friendly, leave off the tomatoes.

1 zucchini, sliced into 8 pieces

1 yellow squash, sliced into 8 pieces

1 cucumber, sliced into 8 pieces

8 cherry tomatoes

8 steamed broccoli florets

8 cauliflower florets

1. On a wooden skewer, thread 1 zucchini slice, 1 yellow squash slice, 1 cucumber slice, 1 cherry tomato, 1 broccoli floret, and 1 cauliflower floret. Set aside.
2. Repeat the process with all remaining ingredients.
3. Serve and eat.

Serves 2. Prep time: 5 minutes

PER SERVING (4 SALAD SKEWERS): CALORIES: 142 / TOTAL FAT: 1.5G / CARBOHYDRATES: 31.2G / FIBER: 8.9G / PROTEIN: 7.8G

SOUTH-OF-THE-BORDER SALAD

QUICK
& EASY

IMMUNITY
BOOST

KIDNEY
SUPPORT

This salad is hearty enough to eat as a main course, or serve alongside one of the other Mexican-inspired dishes in this book. Although corn is a staple in much Mexican food, it is on the "No Go" list. You won't even miss it here. The fresh cilantro is the key to making this salad bright and delicious. Serve it with the Cilantro Salad Dressing (page 208), if desired.

Recipe Tip Feel free to add any other vegetables you might like, such as shredded carrot or sliced jicama.

5 cups chopped romaine lettuce

½ cup sprouted black beans (see page 201)

1 cup cherry tomatoes, halved

1 avocado, diced

¼ cup chopped almonds

½ cup chopped fresh cilantro

½ cup Salsa Fresca (page 198)

1. In a large bowl, add the lettuce, beans, tomatoes, avocado, almonds, cilantro, and Salsa Fresca. Toss all ingredients to combine.
2. Divide the salad evenly between two bowls and serve.

Serves 2. Prep time: 15 minutes

PER SERVING (ABOUT 4 CUPS): CALORIES: 370 / TOTAL FAT: 16.9G / CARBOHYDRATES: 44.3G / FIBER: 14.1G / PROTEIN: 15.3G

ROASTED VEGETABLE SALAD

QUICK
& EASY

IMMUNITY
BOOST

KIDNEY
SUPPORT

This is the perfect way to use up leftover vegetables after a barbecue. If you don't have any, simply roast some vegetables specifically for this dish. Doing so adds a smoky, sweet flavor to the salad. And, as usual, feel free to use any vegetables you have on hand. Remember, if you're on the Thyroid-Support Plan, omit the cherry tomatoes called for in this salad.

Recipe Tip This is another one of those dishes that's great to have on hand. You can use these roasted vegetables for smoothies, soups, wraps, or stir-fries.

½ bunch asparagus, trimmed

1 pint cherry tomatoes

½ cup mushrooms, halved

1 carrot, peeled and cut into
   bite-size pieces

1 red or yellow bell pepper, seeded and cut
   into bite-size pieces

1 tablespoon coconut oil

1 tablespoon garlic powder

1 teaspoon sea salt

1. Preheat the oven to 425°F.
2. In a bowl, add the asparagus, tomatoes, mushrooms, carrot, and bell pepper. Add the coconut oil, garlic powder, and salt. Toss to coat the vegetables evenly.
3. Transfer the vegetables to a baking pan, place in the preheated oven, and roast for 15 minutes, or until the vegetables are tender.
4. Transfer the vegetables to a large bowl. Refrigerate, if desired.
5. Divide the vegetables into two bowls and serve either warm or cold.

Serves 2. Prep time: 10 minutes. Cook time: 15 minutes

PER SERVING (1 CUP): CALORIES: 132 / TOTAL FAT: 7.3G / CARBOHYDRATES: 15.4G / FIBER: 4.2G / PROTEIN: 2.9G

PAD THAI SALAD

QUICK
& EASY

IMMUNITY
BOOST

THYROID
SUPPORT

KIDNEY
SUPPORT

Traditional Pad Thai is a stir-fried dish made with rice noodles, eggs, tamarind, and fish sauce, and is often served with chicken or shrimp. Clearly, most of those ingredients aren't alkaline friendly, but this salad has the same great flavors with none of the bad stuff.

Recipe Tip The bean sprouts called for here are the traditional ones. They are found in the produce section of your market. Alternatively, you can use the thinner alfalfa sprouts. Sprouts are a super alkaline food. Also, look for tamarind paste in the international food section of your market.

4 cups chopped iceberg lettuce

1 cup bean sprouts

2 carrots, cut into thin slices or spirals

1 zucchini, cut into thin strips or spirals

1 scallion, finely chopped

2 tablespoons chopped almonds

Juice of 1 lime

1 garlic clove

1 teaspoon tamarind paste

1 packet stevia

½ teaspoon sea salt

1. In a large bowl, combine the lettuce, bean sprouts, carrots, zucchini, scallion, and almonds.
2. In a small food processor bowl, add the lime juice, garlic, tamarind, stevia, and salt. Blend to combine.
3. Pour the dressing over the vegetables and mix thoroughly.
4. Divide evenly between two bowls and serve.

Serves 2. Prep time: 10 minutes

PER SERVING (ABOUT 3 CUPS): CALORIES: 77 / TOTAL FAT: 3.2G / CARBOHYDRATES: 6.4G / FIBER: 5.5G / PROTEIN: 2G

QUICK
& EASY

IMMUNITY
BOOST

KIDNEY
SUPPORT

QUINOA AND AVOCADO SALAD

This power salad packs nutrition and flavor. The quinoa adds a crunchy, nutty flavor and is a great source of protein. The avocado adds a creamy balance, and contributes healthy fats. Round out the salad with some tomatoes and cucumbers, and you have a hearty, satisfying meal that will leave you feeling great. You can even use this as a filling for the Salad in Your Hand (page 119). Omit the cherry tomatoes if you're following the Thyroid-Support Plan.

Recipe Tip To make this a dish for a holiday party, use red quinoa. The red and green colors will be festive complements to any seasonal buffet.

1 cup cooked quinoa, cooled

1 avocado, cut into cubes

1 cup cherry tomatoes, halved

1 cup cucumber, peeled and diced

¼ cup chopped cilantro

1 tablespoon garlic powder

1 tablespoon onion powder

1 teaspoon sea salt

1 tablespoon freshly squeezed lemon juice

1. In a large bowl, stir together the quinoa, avocado, tomatoes, cucumber, cilantro, garlic powder, onion powder, salt, and lemon juice.
2. Chill for 15 minutes to allow the flavors to blend.
3. Serve immediately, or keep refrigerated for 2 to 3 days.

Serves 2. Prep time: 10 minutes

PER SERVING (ABOUT 2 CUPS): CALORIES: 433 / TOTAL FAT: 14.8G / CARBOHYDRATES: 63.6G / FIBER: 9.9G / PROTEIN: 13.7G

AVOCADO–CAPRESE SALAD

QUICK
& EASY

IMMUNITY
BOOST

KIDNEY
SUPPORT

This might just be the simplest recipe in the entire book! A traditional caprese salad is simply layers of sliced mozzarella, tomatoes, and basil, drizzled with extra-virgin olive oil and sprinkled with salt. Here, the cheese is replaced with avocado, and the oil has been eliminated. This salad is as beautiful as it is easy and healthy.

Recipe Tip If you can't find heirloom tomatoes, use another large tomato. But if tomatoes aren't in season, save this recipe for a time when they are. They are the star!

2 large heirloom tomatoes, sliced

1 avocado, sliced

1 bunch basil leaves

1 teaspoon sea salt

1. On a platter, layer 1 tomato slice, 1 avocado slice, and 1 basil leaf. Repeat the pattern with all remaining tomato slices, avocado slices, and basil leaves.
2. Season with the salt and serve.

Serves 2. Prep time: 5 minutes

PER SERVING (½ FINISHED RECIPE): CALORIES: 125 / TOTAL FAT: 10.1G /
CARBOHYDRATES: 9.1G / FIBER: 4.9G / PROTEIN: 2G

QUICK
& EASY

IMMUNITY
BOOST

THYROID
SUPPORT

KIDNEY
SUPPORT

SPICY SESAME NOODLE SALAD

As with all the noodle recipes in this book, this one is made by substituting vegetables for the noodles. Spaghetti squash stands in here as a healthy alternative to rice or wheat noodles in this tasty dish. And, the spicy sesame dressing will make it so you don't even notice the difference! Serve this salad warm or cool.

Recipe Tip This recipe is great with shredded Chinese cabbage instead of the spaghetti squash. But you'll need to let it sit in the dressing for an hour or so before serving for the cabbage to soften.

1 roasted spaghetti squash
  (see note, below)
2 cups cooked broccoli florets
1 red bell pepper, seeded and cut
  into strips

1 scallion, chopped
1 tablespoon sesame oil
1 teaspoon red pepper flakes
1 teaspoon sea salt
2 tablespoons toasted sesame seeds

1. Prepare the spaghetti squash "noodles" by removing the inside of the cooked squash with a fork into a large bowl.
2. Add the broccoli, red bell pepper, and scallion.
3. In a small bowl, combine the sesame oil, red pepper flakes, and salt. Drizzle atop the vegetables. Toss gently to combine.
4. Garnish with the sesame seeds and serve.

To roast a spaghetti squash, cut the squash in half lengthwise and scrape out the seeds. Brush each half with 2 tablespoons of coconut oil and season with 1 teaspoon of sea salt. Place the squash halves cut-side up on a baking sheet and roast at 350°F for about 50 minutes, or until fork tender.

Serves 4. Prep time: 10 minutes

PER SERVING (1 CUP): CALORIES: 111 / TOTAL FAT: 6G / CARBOHYDRATES: 6.4G /
FIBER: 2.5G / PROTEIN: 2.5G

SPICY ORANGE–BROCCOLI SALAD

QUICK
& EASY

IMMUNITY
BOOST

THYROID
SUPPORT

KIDNEY
SUPPORT

This salad is so simple and elegant you could serve it to company. Or, you could eat it standing in front of your open refrigerator at 11 pm. The combination of broccoli and orange is classic. This vitamin-rich high-fiber salad goes well with just about any other dish in this cookbook. Just don't forget to close the refrigerator door when you're done.

Recipe Tip Stir-fry this salad and eat it warm for a hearty meal.

4 cups cooked broccoli florets, cooled

2 seedless tangerines, peeled and
  separated

⅓ cup freshly squeezed orange juice

2 tablespoons sesame oil

2 garlic cloves, minced

½ teaspoon sea salt

¼ teaspoon red pepper flakes

1. In a large bowl, combine the broccoli and tangerine sections.
2. In a blender, combine the orange juice, sesame oil, garlic, salt, and red pepper flakes. Blend until smooth.
3. Pour the dressing over the broccoli salad. Refrigerate for 1 hour to blend the flavors.
4. Serve cold.

Serves 4. Prep time: 5 minutes

PER SERVING (1 ¼ CUPS): CALORIES: 103 / TOTAL FAT: 7.2G / CARBOHYDRATES: 13.7G / FIBER: 3.5G / PROTEIN: 2.8G

QUICK
& EASY

IMMUNITY
BOOST

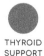

THYROID
SUPPORT

KIDNEY
SUPPORT

WARM SPINACH SALAD

Typically, this salad is served with a very vinegary warm bacon dressing. Instead, this recipe adds shiitake mushrooms for a nice chew and toasted almonds for a warm flavor. Be sure to add the warm dressing right before serving, so the salad doesn't get soggy. Also, baby spinach leaves tend to be more tender than the larger kind.

Recipe Tip Sprinkle some nutritional yeast on the salad to enhance the warm flavor and give yourself a boost of B vitamins.

1 (6-ounce) package baby spinach leaves

½ cup chopped, toasted almonds

1 tablespoon sesame oil

1 tablespoon apple cider vinegar

1 teaspoon sea salt

1 cup chopped shiitake mushrooms

Water, as needed

1. In a large bowl, combine the spinach and almonds.
2. In a small saucepan set over low heat, combine the sesame oil, cider vinegar, salt, and mushrooms. Cook for about 5 minutes, or until the mushrooms soften, adding water if needed.
3. Drizzle the mushroom dressing over the spinach. Toss well to coat the spinach leaves.
4. Serve immediately.

Serves 2. Prep time: 2 minutes. Cook time: 5 minutes

PER SERVING (2 CUPS): CALORIES: 271 / TOTAL FAT: 19.4G / CARBOHYDRATES: 20.3G / FIBER: 7.6G / PROTEIN: 10.2G

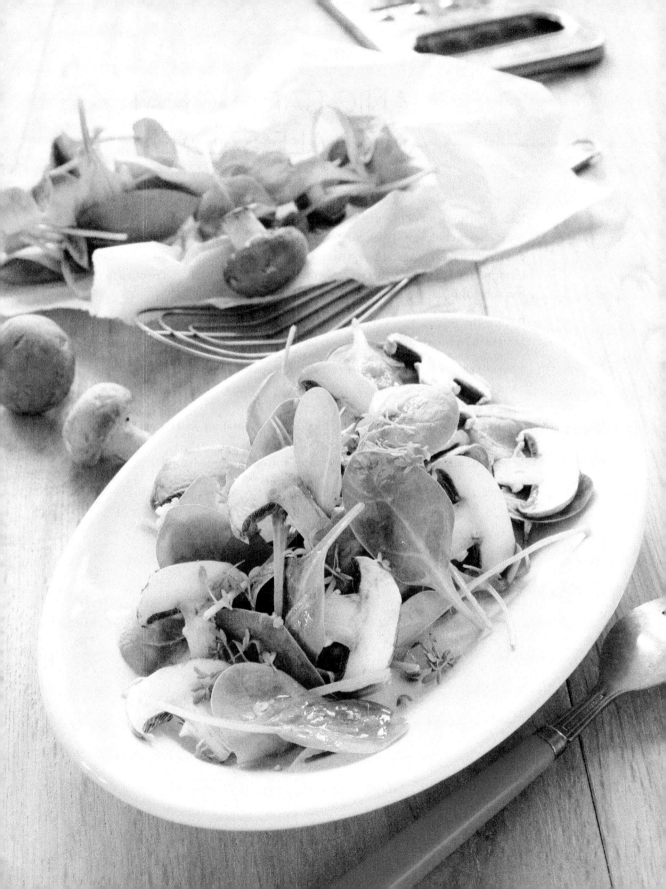

QUICK
& EASY

IMMUNITY
BOOST

KIDNEY
SUPPORT

ORGANIC BABY TOMATO AND KALE SALAD

Kale is getting a lot of press these days as a superfood. And, considering that experts say it lowers cholesterol, helps detoxify the body, and can reduce the risk of five different types of cancers, it's no wonder. Kale can be a bit bitter. The stems are the bitter part, which is why this recipe only calls for the leaves. If you're not a fan, you can substitute lettuce for half of the kale.

Recipe Tip Be sure to wash the kale thoroughly. Like most leafy greens, it can have sand in it. Nothing ruins a great salad faster than biting down on gritty sand.

1 bunch kale, stemmed, leaves washed and chopped

2 cups organic baby tomatoes

2 tablespoons Ranch Dressing (page 211)

1. In a large bowl, toss together the kale leaves, tomatoes, and Ranch Dressing until the dressing thoroughly coats the leaves.
2. Divide equally onto two serving plates and enjoy immediately.

Serves 2. Prep time: 10 minutes

PER SERVING (2 CUPS): CALORIES: 58 / TOTAL FAT: 6.9G / CARBOHYDRATES: 1.6G / FIBER: 6.8G / PROTEIN: 1.1G

EMERALD FOREST SALAD

QUICK
& EASY

IMMUNITY
BOOST

THYROID
SUPPORT

KIDNEY
SUPPORT

For generations, children have referred to broccoli as trees. In this salad, broccoli trees are combined with asparagus spears to make a salad that Jack would be proud to eat from his beanstalk. Cooked quinoa represents the forest floor in this whimsical meal. This salad also makes an excellent filling for a Salad in Your Hand (page 119).

Recipe Tip When choosing asparagus, the thinner the spears, the milder the flavor. Also, white asparagus has a very mild taste.

1 cup cooked broccoli florets, roughly chopped

1 cup trimmed and cooked asparagus spears, roughly chopped

2 cups cooked quinoa, cooled

½ cup water

2 tablespoons freshly squeezed lemon juice

2 tablespoons coconut oil

½ teaspoon sea salt

1. In a large bowl, combine the broccoli and asparagus.
2. Stir in the quinoa.
3. In a blender, combine the water, lemon juice, coconut oil, and salt. Blend until the ingredients emulsify. Pour the dressing over the salad. Stir to combine.
4. Refrigerate the salad for 15 minutes to chill.
5. Serve cold.

Serves 4. Prep time: 5 minutes

PER SERVING (1 CUP): CALORIES: 364 / TOTAL FAT: 11.8G / CARBOHYDRATES: 53G / FIBER: 6.2G / PROTEIN: 12.2G

ASIAN CABBAGE SLAW

QUICK
& EASY

IMMUNITY
BOOST

THYROID
SUPPORT

KIDNEY
SUPPORT

Traditional cole slaw is laden with greasy mayonnaise, rendering it off-limits for anyone interested in healthy eating. This version has an Asian flair. Serve alongside any of the Asian recipes in this cookbook, or eat a big bowl of it all by itself for lunch. The combination of red and green cabbage boosts the nutrition and makes for a beautiful presentation.

Recipe Tip Add some sliced scallions or Mandarin oranges for an added flavor boost.

2 cups shredded green cabbage

2 cups shredded purple cabbage

½ cup sliced, toasted almonds

½ teaspoon sea salt

¼ cup Asian Citrus Dressing (page 209)

1. In a bowl, combine the green cabbage, purple cabbage, almonds, and salt.
2. Add the dressing and mix well. Serve.

Serves 4. Prep time: 5 minutes

PER SERVING (1 CUP): CALORIES: 119 / TOTAL FAT: 5.3G / CARBOHYDRATES: 17.6G / FIBER: 2.6G / PROTEIN: 3.9G

RUSSIAN RUBY SALAD

This is a gorgeous salad. It uses ruby red beets, golden beets, and carrots for a color explosion. You can adjust the size easily by doubling or tripling the recipe. The earthiness of the beets and the sweetness of the carrots and raisins make this a delicious treat.

Recipe Tip Did you know that you could buy purple and red carrots? Visiting a farmers' market or organic farm can open up a whole new world to differently colored vegetables. Feel free to experiment in this colorful salad.

1 red beet, peeled and shredded

1 golden beet, peeled and shredded

2 carrots, peeled and shredded

2 tablespoons hazelnuts

2 tablespoons golden raisins

½ teaspoon sea salt

1. In a medium bowl, stir together the red beet, golden beet, carrots, hazelnuts, golden raisins, and salt.
2. Refrigerate for 15 minutes to blend the flavors. Serve.

Serves 2. Prep time: 15 minutes

PER SERVING (1 CUP): CALORIES: 101 / TOTAL FAT: 0.3G / CARBOHYDRATES: 25.3G / FIBER: 3.2G / PROTEIN: 1.9G

QUICK
& EASY

IMMUNITY
BOOST

KIDNEY
SUPPORT

AVOCADO, STRAWBERRY, SPINACH SALAD

This salad just screams summertime. And with fresh, ripe strawberries, it's no wonder. If strawberries aren't in season, pick another salad to make. It's just not the same unless the strawberries are juicy and sweet. Also, choose avocados that are firm, but not hard or mushy.

Recipe Tip To keep the other half of the avocado from turning brown, leave the pit in and wrap it with plastic wrap before refrigerating.

4 cups baby spinach

1 cup fresh strawberries, sliced

½ cup whole raw almonds

½ avocado, diced

¼ cup Avocado Salad Dressing (page 210)

1. In a large bowl, combine the spinach, strawberries, almonds, avocado, and dressing. Toss well to coat the salad evenly.
2. Serve immediately.

Serves 4. Prep time: 5 minutes

PER SERVING (1½ CUPS): CALORIES: 117 / TOTAL FAT: 8.7G / CARBOHYDRATES: 8.3G / FIBER: 3.7G / PROTEIN: 4G

SUMMER DINNER SALAD

QUICK
& EASY

IMMUNITY
BOOST

KIDNEY
SUPPORT

This basic salad can be adapted to include whatever vegetables you have on hand, and it's perfect for a hot summer night when you don't want to cook. Just toss everything together with your favorite dressing from chapter 11 (page 195) and serve. And a reminder, if you're on the Thyroid-Support Plan, remember to omit the cherry tomatoes called for here.

Recipe Tip This salad can be made with any kind of lettuce. Experiment with mixed greens or some other variety you haven't tried before.

4 cups chopped iceberg or
  romaine lettuce

2 cups cherry tomatoes, halved

1 (14.5-ounce) can whole green
  beans, drained

½ cup shredded carrot

1 scallion, sliced

1 cucumber, peeled and sliced

2 radishes, thinly sliced

1. In a large bowl, combine the lettuce, tomatoes, green beans, carrot, scallion, cucumber, and radishes.
2. Toss well with 2 tablespoons of your dressing of choice and serve immediately.

Serves 4. Prep time: 5 minutes

PER SERVING (2 CUPS, WITHOUT DRESSING): CALORIES: 39 / TOTAL FAT: 0.3G / CARBOHYDRATES: 9G / FIBER: 2.1G / PROTEIN: 1.6G

UNDER-THE-SEA SALAD

QUICK
& EASY

IMMUNITY
BOOST

THYROID
SUPPORT

KIDNEY
SUPPORT

This salad is not going to be for everyone. But, it contains a lot of foods known to be super alkaline and is incredibly high in trace minerals like iodine and iron—things that the body really needs. Even if you're not sure you'll like it, try it once. You might find you love these oceanic delights!

Recipe Tip You can find sea vegetables and seaweed in a health food store (sometimes you can even find seaweed in your regular grocery store). You can also find sea vegetables online in the Resources section.

1 cup dried sea vegetables

1 ounce dry seaweed

1 teaspoon spirulina

1 teaspoon apple cider vinegar

1 packet stevia

1 teaspoon sesame seeds

1. Reconstitute the dried sea vegetables and seaweed according to the package directions.
2. Meanwhile, in a small bowl, mix together the spirulina, cider vinegar, and stevia.
3. Drain the sea vegetables and seaweed. Squeeze any excess moisture from them and place them in a medium bowl. Add the spirulina mixture and toss to combine.
4. Refrigerate for 1 hour to blend the flavors.
5. Top with the sesame seeds and serve.

Serves 2. Prep time: 5 minutes

PER SERVING (1 CUP): CALORIES: 61 / TOTAL FAT: 0.2G / CARBOHYDRATES: 4.1G / FIBER: 6.5G / PROTEIN: 2.3G

MARINATED VEGETABLES

This is a classic deli salad, but in this version the acid-producing oil and vinegar are replaced with healthier alternatives. Since there are some beans in this recipe, consider it part of your 20 percent. Chill this salad overnight so the flavors can meld.

Recipe Tip To lower the acidity of this dish even more (so you can eat it more often), sprout your beans and use them in place of the canned kidney beans. Just sprout 2 cups of dried beans (see page 201) and enjoy this meal as often as you like!

1 (14.5-ounce) can whole green
  beans, drained

1 (16-ounce) can kidney beans

1 (14.5-ounce) can carrots (or 2 cups
  steamed fresh carrots)

1 cup button mushrooms

1 (4-ounce) jar pimiento peppers, drained

1 cup water

¼ cup coconut oil

¼ cup apple cider vinegar

2 tablespoons dried oregano

1 tablespoon garlic powder

1 tablespoon onion powder

1 teaspoon sea salt

1. In a medium bowl, combine the green beans, kidney beans, carrots, mushrooms, and pimientos.
2. In a blender, add the water, coconut oil, cider vinegar, oregano, garlic powder, onion powder, and salt. Blend to emulsify the ingredients.
3. Pour the dressing over the vegetables. Toss to combine. Cover and chill overnight.

Serves 4. Prep time: 5 minutes

PER SERVING (1 CUP): CALORIES: 198 / TOTAL FAT: 9.7G / CARBOHYDRATES: 11.1G /
FIBER: 3.5G / PROTEIN: 2.5G

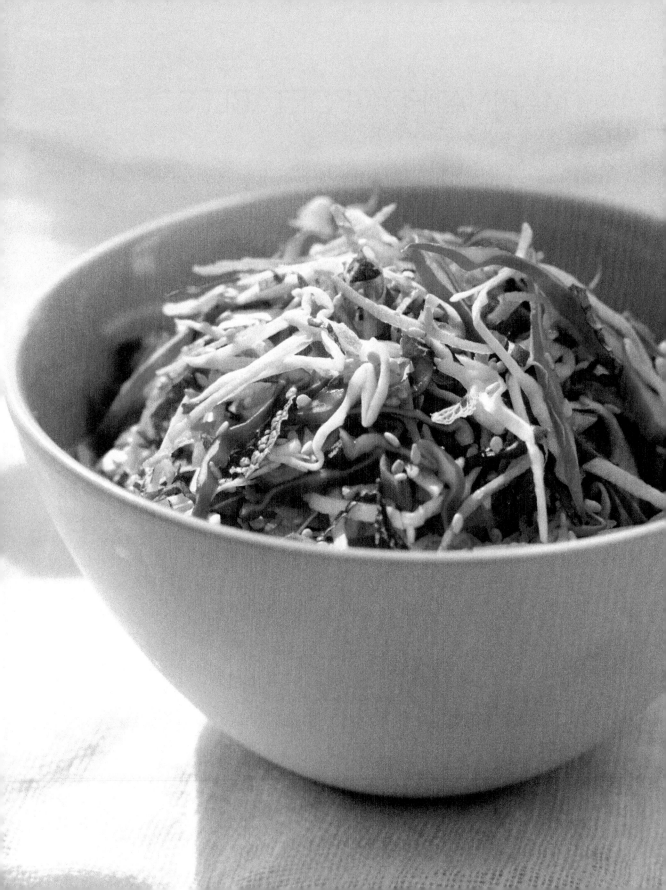

8

BOUNTIFUL BOWLS

THE ASIAN BOWL

QUICK
& EASY

IMMUNITY
BOOST

THYROID
SUPPORT

KIDNEY
SUPPORT

This first recipe in this bowl chapter is a good illustration of the basics of bowl assembly. The standard way to make a good bowl is to layer a grain, a bean, a vegetable, and a sauce. Of course, the recipes in this book only include ingredients on the approved food list, so grains often are replaced with another vegetable. The base for this Asian Bowl is shredded cabbage. If you're in the mood for a warm bowl, sauté the cabbage and carrots first.

Recipe Tip Cashew butter is usually located near the peanut butter in grocery stores. If you can't find cashew butter, you can use almond butter; just make sure it doesn't have added sugar.

1 cup shredded green cabbage

1 cup shredded red cabbage

1 cup chopped carrots

¼ cup water chestnuts

3 tablespoons chopped scallions

1 tablespoon dark sesame oil

1 tablespoon cashew butter

¼ teaspoon red pepper flakes, or additional as needed

½ teaspoon ginger powder

Hot water, as needed

2 teaspoons toasted sesame seeds

1. In a medium bowl, layer the green and red cabbage, then the carrots, water chestnuts, and scallions.
2. In a blender, add the sesame oil, cashew butter, red pepper flakes, and ginger powder. Blend until the ingredients emulsify. Add hot water, by the teaspoon, if the dressing is too thick.
3. Pour the dressing over the vegetables, add sesame seeds, and serve.

Serves 1. Prep time: 5 minutes

PER SERVING: CALORIES: 317 / TOTAL FAT: 24.7G / CARBOHYDRATES: 20.8G /
FIBER: 6.6G / PROTEIN: 7.2G

THE BREAKUP BOWL

QUICK
& EASY

IMMUNITY
BOOST

THYROID
SUPPORT

KIDNEY
SUPPORT

It's happened to almost everyone. You get dumped. Don't let that derail your healthy eating plan! Instead of crying over a pint of ice cream, dump these sweet, healthy ingredients into a bowl and soothe your body and your soul.

Recipe Tip You can add other fruits as you like. Frozen cherries are a great addition, as are fresh strawberries.

2 bananas, peeled, sliced, and frozen

2 tablespoons coconut milk

2 tablespoons fruit-sweetened-only
  strawberry jam

2 tablespoons grated unsweetened coconut

2 tablespoons chopped toasted almonds

¼ cup Coconut Whipped Cream (page 202)

1. In a food processor, place the frozen bananas. Add the coconut milk and blend until they're the consistency of ice cream. Transfer to a single-serving bowl.
2. Top the bananas with the jam, coconut, toasted almonds, and whipped cream.
3. Serve immediately.

Serves 1. Prep time: 5 minutes

PER SERVING: CALORIES: 454 / TOTAL FAT: 19.2G / CARBOHYDRATES: 69.4G / FIBER: 9.6G / PROTEIN: 6.9G

THE COMFORT BOWL

QUICK
& EASY

IMMUNITY
BOOST

THYROID
SUPPORT

KIDNEY
SUPPORT

This bowl is perfect for when you've had a bad day. Curl up on the couch with this heartwarming—and healthy—dish. This is the only recipe in the book that uses mashed potatoes. Because of this, it should be considered part of your 20 percent.

Recipe Tip Depending on whether you like peas, you may not find them comforting. If not, then substitute an alkaline-friendly vegetable that does comfort you, like maybe spinach or lima beans.

1 cup cooked baby potatoes

2 tablespoons almond milk

½ teaspoon sea salt

½ cup green peas

½ cup Great Gravy (page 200)

1. In a medium bowl, combine the potatoes, almond milk, and salt. Mash with a fork to the desired consistency.
2. Top the potatoes with the peas and the gravy. Warm the bowl in the microwave on high for 1 minute, and eat.

Serves 1. Prep time: 15 minutes

PER SERVING: CALORIES: 205 / TOTAL FAT: 2.4G / CARBOHYDRATES: 41.3G /
FIBER: 7.3G / PROTEIN: 8.1G

QUICK
& EASY

IMMUNITY
BOOST

THYROID
SUPPORT

KIDNEY
SUPPORT

THE FIGHT IT OFF BOWL

This bowl is kind of cheating, because it's basically a soup. But, it's a great choice when you think you're fighting off a cold or the flu. Make a big bowl of this nutritious concoction, and show those germs that you're the boss. Your immune system will thank you.

Recipe Tip Add other vegetables to boost the healing properties. If you're going to use spinach, though, add it no more than 5 minutes before serving.

2 cups vegetable broth

1 carrot, peeled and sliced

½ cup bite-size broccoli florets

2 garlic cloves, finely minced

1. In a medium saucepan set over medium heat, combine the broth, carrot, broccoli, and garlic. Cook for 10 minutes, or until vegetables reach a desired level of tenderness.
2. Pour into a bowl, and eat.

Serves 1. Prep time: 5 minutes. Cook time: 10 minutes

PER SERVING: CALORIES: 126 / TOTAL FAT: 2.9G / CARBOHYDRATES: 12.8G /
FIBER: 2.8G / PROTEIN: 11.8G

THE HARVEST BOWL

QUICK
& EASY

IMMUNITY
BOOST

THYROID
SUPPORT

KIDNEY
SUPPORT

This recipe is like Thanksgiving in a bowl, but instead of acid-producing turkey and stuffing, this bowl offers the best of the autumn harvest. The combination of wild rice, apples, sweet potatoes, and gravy are classic and delicious.

Recipe Tip Add some green beans or mushrooms, for extra nutrition and flavor. Maybe both!

1 cup cooked brown rice

¼ cup cooked wild rice

1 apple, peeled, cored, and diced

½ cup mashed sweet potato

¼ cup Great Gravy (page 200)

1. In a medium bowl, layer the brown rice, wild rice, apple, sweet potato, and gravy.
2. Microwave on high for about 2 minutes, or until warm. Serve.

Serves 1. Prep time: 10 minutes

PER SERVING: CALORIES: 579 / TOTAL FAT: 3.1G / CARBOHYDRATES: 45.7G /

FIBER: 3.6G / PROTEIN: 8.9G

THE HAWAIIAN BOWL

QUICK
& EASY

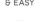

IMMUNITY
BOOST

THYROID
SUPPORT

KIDNEY
SUPPORT

This recipe is one of the few in this book that calls for brown rice. Since it's on the limit list, this bowl should be considered one of your 20 percent meals. The Home-made Barbecue Sauce that tops this is so delicious you might want to top everything with it. Feel free to add different vegetables, as you choose.

Recipe Tip The sauce will keep for a few days in the refrigerator, or you can freeze it and it will last for months.

To render this recipe a choice for the Thyroid-Support Plan, substitute the Asian Citrus Dressing (page 209) for the Homemade Barbecue Sauce used here.

½ cup cooked brown rice

1 cup steamed broccoli

¼ cup packed-in-juice pineapple chunks,
  drained, liquid reserved

2 tablespoons Homemade Barbecue Sauce
  (page 207)

1. In a medium bowl, layer the brown rice, broccoli, and pineapple.
2. In a small saucepan set over medium heat, whisk together the reserved pineapple juice and the Homemade Barbecue Sauce for about 5 minutes, until thickened and bubbly.
3. Pour over the rice and broccoli and serve.

Serves 1. Prep time: 5 minutes. Cook time: 5 minutes

PER SERVING: CALORIES: 223 / TOTAL FAT: 1.6G / CARBOHYDRATES: 47.6G /
FIBER: 4.6G / PROTEIN: 3.6G

THE HOLLYWOOD BOWL

QUICK
& EASY

IMMUNITY
BOOST

THYROID
SUPPORT

KIDNEY
SUPPORT

What do you think of when you think of Hollywood? Stars! This bowl is made with star-shaped food, so you'll need a star-shaped cookie cutter. The recipe also calls for a star fruit that, when cut, is naturally in the shape of a star.

Recipe Tip Even if you don't cut the watermelon into star shapes, this is a delicious bowl. After all, Hollywood stars make their own rules!

1 star fruit

¼ watermelon, cut into slices

¼ cup Coconut Whipped Cream (page 202)

1. Slice the star fruit into star-shaped pieces.
2. Press the cookie cutter into watermelon slices to create star-shaped pieces.
3. Add the star fruit and watermelon to a single-serving bowl. Top with the Coconut Whipped Cream.
4. Serve immediately.

Serves 1. Prep time: 5 minutes

PER SERVING: CALORIES: 125 / TOTAL FAT: 9.6G / CARBOHYDRATES: 9.3G /

FIBER: 2.7G / PROTEIN: 1.8G

THE INDIAN BOWL

QUICK
& EASY

IMMUNITY
BOOST

KIDNEY
SUPPORT

This delicious bowl starts with a layer of nutty, crunchy quinoa. It's topped with just a few chickpeas, then a layer of steamed vegetables. Finally, a delicious coconut curry sauce drenches this bowl in creamy goodness.

Recipe Tip For a change of pace, add some eggplant, too. Just remember that doing so will make this unsuitable for those on the Thyroid-Support Plan.

1 cup cooked quinoa, warmed

1 large carrot, peeled, sliced, and steamed

½ cup cooked cauliflower florets

⅛ cup chickpeas

¼ cup sliced mushrooms

½ cup coconut milk

1 tablespoon yellow curry powder

½ teaspoon ground ginger

1 teaspoon sea salt

1 tablespoon tomato paste

1. In a medium bowl, layer the quinoa, carrot, cauliflower, and chickpeas.
2. In a small saucepan set over medium heat, combine the mushrooms, coconut milk, curry powder, ginger, salt, and tomato paste. Whisk until the mixture simmers. Cook for 5 minutes and then cool slightly.
3. Pour the sauce over the quinoa mixture and serve immediately.

Serves 1. Prep time: 10 minutes. Cook time: 5 minutes

PER SERVING: CALORIES: 469 / TOTAL FAT: 0.2G / CARBOHYDRATES: 26.1G / FIBER: 13.5G / PROTEIN: 5.4G

THE ITALIAN BOWL

QUICK
& EASY

IMMUNITY
BOOST

KIDNEY
SUPPORT

This recipe has all the classic Italian flavors without the fat-laden meats and sausage. Once you've made this once or twice, feel free to play around with the ingredients. Add bell peppers for sweetness, green beans or broccoli for more vegetables, or any garden vegetables you have on hand. Be sure to use fresh herbs, as they add the bright flavor to this dish.

Recipe Tip Make a double batch and combine the ingredients in a pot with 2 cups of vegetable broth to make a hearty Italian soup. Warm over medium heat and serve hot.

1 (14.5-ounce) can tomatoes, whole, diced, or crushed, undrained

1 medium onion, diced

½ cup sliced zucchini

4 garlic cloves, minced

⅓ cup fresh chopped basil

½ teaspoon chopped fresh oregano

2 tablespoons freshly squeezed lemon juice

1 cup cooked quinoa, warmed

½ cup eggplant, peeled, diced, cooked, and rewarmed

1. Drain 2 tablespoons of liquid from the tomatoes and add it to a medium saucepan set over medium heat. Add the onion and sauté for 5 minutes, or until translucent.
2. Add the tomatoes with their remaining juices, zucchini, garlic, basil, and oregano. Stir to combine. Simmer for 5 minutes. Remove from the heat and stir in the lemon juice.
3. In a single-serving bowl, layer the quinoa and the eggplant. Top with the tomato mixture.
4. Serve warm.

Serves 1. Prep time: 5 minutes. Cook time: 10 minutes

PER SERVING: CALORIES: 390 / TOTAL FAT: 5.4G / CARBOHYDRATES: 71.5G / FIBER: 10.8G / PROTEIN: 14.5G

QUICK
& EASY

IMMUNITY
BOOST

KIDNEY
SUPPORT

THE LADY AND THE TRAMP BOWL

This bowl is named after the classic scene in the movie *Lady and the Tramp* where the two characters share a bowl of pasta and end up kissing. As such, this is the only bowl in the chapter that serves two—kissing optional. Spaghetti squash stands in for the pasta in this dish. A layer of fresh tomatoes and a topping of Sun-Dried Tomato Sauce (page 204) make this date-worthy.

Recipe Tip Feel free to layer in any additional vegetables that you like. Mushrooms, spinach, or even broccoli would be good.

2 cups cooked, shredded spaghetti squash (see note below)

1 cup chopped fresh tomatoes

1 cup Sun-Dried Tomato Sauce (page 204)

1. Layer the spaghetti squash and tomatoes in a bowl big enough for two people. Top with the Sun-Dried Tomato Sauce.
2. In the microwave, warm the bowl for 2 minutes on high, or until heated through.
3. Serve with two forks and lots of napkins.

To roast a spaghetti squash, cut the squash in half lengthwise and scrape out the seeds. Brush each half with 2 tablespoons of coconut oil and season with 1 teaspoon of sea salt. Place the squash halves cut-side up on a baking sheet and roast at 350°F for about 50 minutes, or until fork tender.

Serves 2. Prep time: 15 minutes

PER SERVING (1½ CUPS PLUS ½ CUP SAUCE): CALORIES: 153 / TOTAL FAT: 4.1G / CARBOHYDRATE: 27.1G / FIBER: 4.2G / PROTEIN: 3.5G

THE LAZY BOWL

QUICK
& EASY

IMMUNITY
BOOST

THYROID
SUPPORT

KIDNEY
SUPPORT

The Lazy Bowl is for those nights when you feel so lazy you don't even have the mojo to cook the simplest dish. This recipe relies on leftovers from other recipes. The formula is simple: Layer 1 is a grain or root vegetable; Layer 2 is a vegetable; Layer 3 is a topping or sauce. The nutritional information is calculated given the sample suggestions. Your results will vary depending on what you include.

Recipe Tip If you know you're going to be super busy one week, make a little extra of everything you cook so you have leftovers on hand to make The Lazy Bowl.

Layer One: 1 cup Baby Potato Home Fries (page 65)

Layer Three: ¼ cup Healthy Hummus (page 103)

Layer Two: ½ cup Marinated Vegetables (page 137)

In a single-serving bowl, layer the potatoes, vegetables, and hummus, and eat!

Serves 1. Prep time: 5 minutes

PER SERVING: CALORIES: 510 / TOTAL FAT: 9.9G / CARBOHYDRATES: 32.4G / FIBER: 6.7G / PROTEIN: 12.8G

QUICK
& EASY

IMMUNITY
BOOST

KIDNEY
SUPPORT

THE MEXICAN BOWL

Who needs to go to a Mexican fast-food restaurant to get a delicious and healthy bowl? Not you! When you make this zesty bowl, you get all the taste and none of the acidifying ingredients that often come with take-out fare. Add a chopped jalapeño if you like things on the spicy side.

Recipe Tip To make this thyroid friendly, omit the salsa.

1 cup sprouted black beans (see page 201)
1 teaspoon ground cumin
1 medium sweet potato, cooked and diced
½ cup chopped cilantro

½ avocado, diced
3 tablespoons Salsa Fresca (page 198)
Pinch sea salt

1. In a small bowl, combine the beans and the cumin.
2. In a medium microwaveable bowl, layer the sweet potatoes and top with the beans. Warm the vegetables in the microwave on high for 2 minutes, or until heated through.
3. Remove from the microwave and layer on the cilantro and avocado, and top with the Salsa Fresca.
4. Season with the salt and serve immediately.

Serves 1. Prep time: 10 minutes

PER SERVING: CALORIES: 436 / TOTAL FAT: 11.4G / CARBOHYDRATES: 69.5G / FIBER: 17.4G / PROTEIN: 17.8G

THE ROSE BOWL

QUICK
& EASY

IMMUNITY
BOOST

THYROID
SUPPORT

KIDNEY
SUPPORT

If life is just a bowl of cherries, then this recipe is full of life! The Rose Bowl contains all red foods in a delicious combination. Red foods contain antioxidants, which help heal the body and prevent disease. They do so by decreasing the inflammation that can cause internal damage.

Recipe Tip If you can't find red quinoa, regular quinoa will work just as well.

1 cup cooked red quinoa

½ cup roasted, diced red peppers

½ cup dark red cherries, pitted and sliced

¾ teaspoon red curry paste

½ cup coconut milk

1. In a single-serving bowl, layer the quinoa, red peppers, and cherries.
2. In a blender, mix together the curry paste and coconut milk. Pour the liquid over the layered quinoa, peppers, and cherries.
3. Microwave on high for about 2 minutes, or until warm.

Serves 1. Prep time: 5 minutes

PER SERVING: CALORIES: 401 / TOTAL FAT: 1.8G / CARBOHYDRATES: 64.5G /
FIBER: 6.7G / PROTEIN: 16.7G

QUICK
& EASY

IMMUNITY
BOOST

KIDNEY
SUPPORT

THE SOUTHERN BOWL

Eating this bowl will make you feel like you're in the Deep South. With sweet potato, southern greens, and okra, this packs a lot of nutrition into one meal. Greens typically are made with meat, but this version tastes just as great with alkaline-friendly ingredients. Also, if you're not a fan of okra, give it a try in this recipe anyway.

Recipe Tip If you're concerned that the okra will be slimy, use the frozen kind.

¼ cup vegetable broth, divided

¼ sweet onion, chopped

1 garlic clove, finely chopped

½ teaspoon sea salt, divided

4 ounces canned diced tomatoes

1 cup collard greens

1 sliced okra, fresh or frozen

1 sweet potato, peeled and cut into
  bite-size pieces

¼ cup almond milk

1. In a large saucepan set over medium heat, heat 2 tablespoons vegetable broth. Add the onion and sauté for 5 minutes, or until translucent.
2. Add the garlic, ¼ teaspoon salt, tomatoes, the remaining 2 tablespoons broth, collard greens, and okra. Simmer for 30 to 35 minutes, or until tender.
3. Meanwhile, in a medium pot of boiling water, cook the sweet potato pieces for 10 minutes, or until tender. Drain and place in a medium bowl. Add the almond milk and the remaining ¼ teaspoon salt. Using an electric mixer, mash the sweet potatoes.
4. Place the warm mashed sweet potato in a bowl. Top with the collard greens and okra mixture. Finish with any tomato sauce left in the pan.

Serves 1. Prep time: 10 minutes. Cook time: 40 minutes

PER SERVING: CALORIES: 201 / TOTAL FAT: 2.7G / CARBOHYDRATES: 37.5G / FIBER: 7.3G / PROTEIN: 9G

THE SUPER BOWL

QUICK
& EASY

IMMUNITY
BOOST

THYROID
SUPPORT

KIDNEY
SUPPORT

Although this recipe shares a name with a famous football game, it has a slightly different meaning. This bowl contains only foods considered to be superfoods. These nutritional powerhouse foods combine to make this recipe high in protein, vitamins, minerals, and fiber. Choose this bowl if you're fighting off a cold.

Recipe Tip Remember that the stems are the part of the kale that is bitter. If you really hate kale, you can substitute spinach.

1 cup cooked quinoa

1 cup kale, raw, steamed, or sautéed

¼ cup açaí berries

1 tablespoon apple cider vinegar

1 tablespoon coconut oil

¼ teaspoon mustard powder

¼ teaspoon sea salt

Dash garlic powder

Dash onion powder

1. In a single-serving bowl, layer the quinoa and kale.
2. In a blender, blend the açaí berries, cider vinegar, coconut oil, mustard powder, salt, garlic powder, and onion powder until the ingredients emulsify.
3. Pour the dressing over quinoa-kale mixture. Toss and serve.

Serves 1. Prep time: 10 minutes

PER SERVING: CALORIES: 424 / TOTAL FAT: 18.7G / CARBOHYDRATES: 52.3G / FIBER: 5.1G / PROTEIN: 11.6G

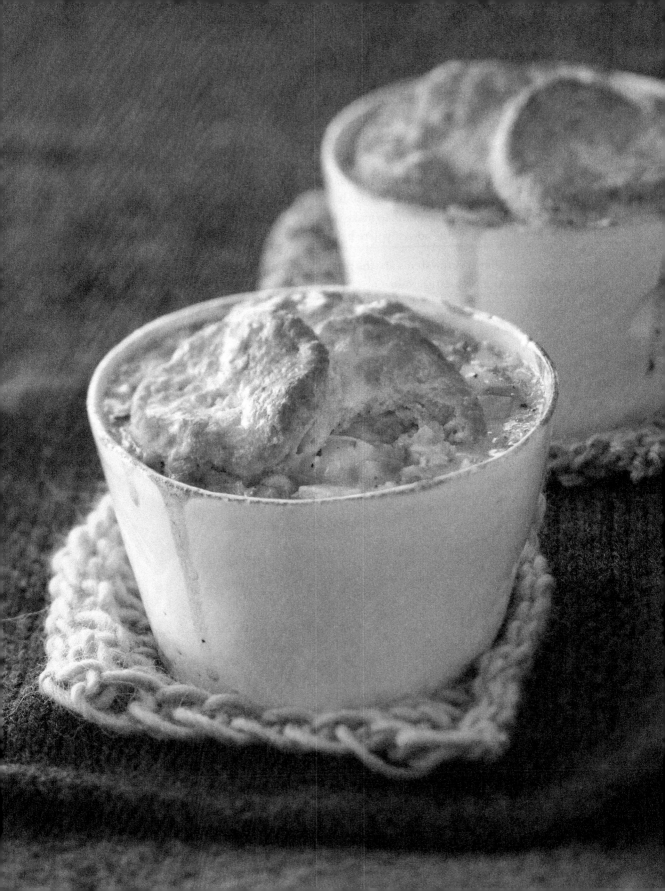

9

MIGHTY
MAIN DISHES

BETTER THAN CHICKEN SOUP

IMMUNITY
BOOST

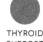

THYROID
SUPPORT

KIDNEY
SUPPORT

There are few things more hearty and satisfying than a bowl of chicken soup. But chicken is on the "No Go" list, so this version uses other savory ingredients. The key to the authentic flavor is in the simmering time. It gives the vegetables and herbs time to blend and settle.

Cooking spray

1 large onion, roughly chopped

2 large carrots, peeled and roughly chopped

2 large celery stalks (with leaves), roughly chopped

1 parsnip, peeled and roughly chopped

5 garlic cloves, smashed

1 leek, cleaned well and roughly chopped

9 cups water

2 bay leaves

2 teaspoons sea salt

1. Spray the bottom of a large stockpot with cooking spray. Place the pot over medium-low heat, add the onion, and sauté for about 5 minutes, stirring constantly.
2. Add the carrots, celery, parsnip, garlic, and leek to the pot. Sauté for another 3 minutes.
3. Add the water, bay leaves, and salt. Simmer for 1 hour.
4. Remove from the heat and cool slightly. Strain out the vegetables, leaving only the broth.
5. To serve, add back some of the vegetables if you wish and warm the soup to the desired temperature.

Serves 4. Prep time: 15 minutes. Cook time: 1 hour, 10 minutes

PER SERVING (2 CUPS): CALORIES: 70 / TOTAL FAT: 0.03G / CARBOHYDRATES: 11.5G / FIBER: 2.2G / PROTEIN: 1.8G

IMMUNITY
BOOST

THYROID
SUPPORT

KIDNEY
SUPPORT

YOU WON'T MISS THE CLAMS CHOWDER

This hearty chowder will surprise you, as it is completely alkaline friendly. The key to a traditional clam chowder is the presence of salty, chewy clams mixed into a thick cream base. In this recipe, we replace the clams with shiitake mushrooms, add some nori seaweed for that ocean flavor, and surround those in a thickened cream-like broth. Make this on those cold, winter days to soothe your heart and health.

For the mushroom clams

½ cup roughly chopped shiitake
 mushrooms

1 teaspoon coconut oil

¼ cup water

½ teaspoon celery seed

For the soup base

½ medium onion, chopped

3 medium carrots, peeled and chopped

2 celery stalks, finely chopped

1 teaspoon dried thyme

3 cups vegetable broth

1 sheet nori, finely crumbled

For the cream base

1 cup lightly steamed cauliflower

¾ cup unsweetened almond milk

¼ teaspoon sea salt

To make the mushroom clams:

1. In a large pot set over medium high heat, add the mushrooms and the coconut oil. Sauté for 3 minutes. Add the water and celery seed, stirring until the water is absorbed.
2. Remove from the heat and transfer the mushrooms to a plate.

To make the soup base:

1. In the same pot over medium heat, sauté the onion, carrots, celery, and thyme for about 5 minutes, or until the onion is softened. Add some of the broth, if needed.
2. Then, add any remaining broth and the nori and bring to a boil.

To make the cream base:

In a blender or food processor, add the cauliflower, almond milk, and salt. Blend to combine. If the mixture is too thick, add some of the soup base to thin. Blend until smooth.

To assemble the chowder:

1. Add the mushroom mix and the cream base to the soup base. Stir well to combine.
2. Heat for 5 minutes, or until warm, and serve.

Serves 4. Prep time: 15 minutes. Cook time: 30 minutes

PER SERVING (1 CUP): CALORIES: 97 / TOTAL FAT: 3.2G / CARBOHYDRATES: 10.8G / FIBER: 2.4G / PROTEIN: 6.5G

QUICK
& EASY

IMMUNITY
BOOST

KIDNEY
SUPPORT

ANGEL HAIR PASTA WITH HEARTY TOMATO SAUCE

This recipe is easy for a quick weeknight meal. Here, spaghetti squash replaces the pasta. And because it uses jarred spaghetti sauce, you get long-simmered flavor in just a few minutes. Be sure to use a sauce that contains no dairy, meat, or added sugar.

¼ onion, chopped

1 teaspoon coconut oil

1 teaspoon sea salt

1 teaspoon minced garlic

½ teaspoon red pepper flakes

1 (6-ounce) can tomato paste

1 (16-ounce) jar spaghetti sauce

½ cup water

2 cups cooked spaghetti squash, shredded into noodles (see note below)

1. In a medium pot set over medium heat, add the onion and coconut oil. Sauté for about 5 minutes, or until tender.
2. Add the salt, garlic, red pepper flakes, and tomato paste. Stir until combined.
3. Add the spaghetti sauce and water. Simmer for 10 minutes.
4. Add the spaghetti squash and stir to combine.
5. Serve immediately.

To roast a spaghetti squash, cut the squash in half lengthwise and scrape out the seeds. Brush each half with 2 tablespoons of coconut oil and season with 1 teaspoon of sea salt. Place the squash halves cut-side up on a baking sheet and roast at 350°F for about 50 minutes, or until fork tender.

Serves 2. Prep time: 15 minutes. Cook time: 15 minutes

PER SERVING (2 CUPS): CALORIES: 284 / TOTAL FAT: 3.8G / CARBOHYDRATES: 36.8G / FIBER: 7.7G / PROTEIN: 8.6G

LOVERS' LASAGNA

IMMUNITY
BOOST

KIDNEY
SUPPORT

Bet you're surprised there's a lasagna recipe in this cookbook! With zucchini strips as the noodles and a delicious White Sauce (page 206), you can have your lasagna and your healthy eating plan, too. The key to great taste is roasting the zucchini for a few minutes so it doesn't make the recipe soggy.

4 zucchini, sliced lengthwise into
  ¼-inch noodles

1 cup Sun-Dried Tomato Sauce (page 204)
1 cup White Sauce (page 206)

1. Preheat the oven to 350°F.
2. Place the zucchini noodles on a baking sheet and into the preheated oven. Roast for 10 minutes, then remove from the oven.
3. In a small lasagna pan, cover the bottom with one layer of zucchini strips. Top that with ¼ cup Sun-Dried Tomato Sauce. Add another layer of zucchini strips, placed crosswise from the first layer. Top with another ¼ cup Sun-Dried Tomato Sauce. Lay a third layer of zucchini crosswise from the second layer and another ¼ cup Sun-Dried Tomato Sauce. Repeat with the remaining zucchini and ¼ cup Sun-Dried Tomato Sauce.
4. Top the finished lasagna with the White Sauce. Cover with aluminum foil, place the pan in the preheated oven, and bake for 15 minutes, or until hot and bubbly.
5. Remove from the oven and cool for 5 minutes before slicing and serving.

Serves 2. Prep time: 10 minutes. Cook time: 25 minutes

PER SERVING (½ FINISHED RECIPE): CALORIES: 184 / TOTAL FAT: 3.6G /
CARBOHYDRATES: 16.1G / FIBER: 4.6G / PROTEIN: 5.4G

STUFFED PEPPERS

QUICK
& EASY

IMMUNITY
BOOST

THYROID
SUPPORT

KIDNEY
SUPPORT

This quick and easy recipe is also very elegant looking. The vibrant peppers combine with the colors of the vegetables and quinoa to make it look restaurant worthy. It's high in fiber, high in protein, and high in deliciousness. The leftovers are a great lunch to take to work the next day, too.

Cooking spray

1 teaspoon coconut oil

½ cup chopped vegetables, zucchini, carrots, or broccoli

1 cup cooked quinoa

1 teaspoon garlic powder

1 teaspoon onion powder

1 teaspoon sea salt

2 bell peppers, any color, cored and seeded; tops removed and reserved

1. Preheat the oven to 350°F.
2. Coat a baking pan with cooking spray.
3. In a medium saucepan set over medium heat, add the coconut oil and chopped vegetables. Sauté for 5 minutes, or until softened.
4. Add the quinoa, garlic powder, onion powder, and salt. Stir to combine.
5. Place each bell pepper upright in the prepared pan. Fill each pepper with one-half of the quinoa-vegetable mix. Top each pepper with its reserved top.
6. Cover with aluminum foil, place in the preheated oven, and bake for 15 minutes, or until the peppers are soft.

Serves 2. Prep time: 5 minutes. Cook time: 20 minutes

PER SERVING (1 STUFFED PEPPER): CALORIES: 213 / TOTAL FAT: 5.1G / CARBOHYDRATES: 34.8G / FIBER: 5.5G / PROTEIN: 7.2G

CURRIED EGGPLANT

QUICK
& EASY

IMMUNITY
BOOST

KIDNEY
SUPPORT

This incredibly easy dish is also healthy and delicious. It's a good idea to keep a broiled eggplant on hand since it's so simple to make, and you'll always have an ingredient on hand to make a quick meal.

1 roasted eggplant, cooled, with contents removed from the shell and reserved

Juice of 1 lemon

1 teaspoon sea salt

1 teaspoon sesame oil

1 teaspoon curry powder

Water, as needed

Cooked quinoa, for serving (optional)

1. In a food processor, combine the eggplant, lemon juice, salt, sesame oil, and curry powder. Blend until smooth.
2. To a small saucepan set over medium heat, transfer the eggplant mixture and warm it for about 5 minutes. Add some water to thin, if necessary.
3. Serve as is, or over quinoa (if using).

To roast eggplant, simply slice it, add a little sea salt, and bake in a 300°F oven for about 30 minutes, or until it's soft. Or, you can roast it whole as called for here, but it will need to cook a bit longer depending on the size, until it's easily pierced with a sharp knife. Refrigerate until ready to use.

Serves 2. Prep time: 5 minutes. Cook time: 5 minutes

PER SERVING (½ FINISHED RECIPE): CALORIES: 81 / TOTAL FAT: 2.8G /
CARBOHYDRATES: 14.1G / FIBER: 8.4G / PROTEIN: 2.4G

CHAMPIONSHIP CHILI

QUICK
& EASY

IMMUNITY
BOOST

KIDNEY
SUPPORT

Few things are better for watching the game than a big bowl of chili. This version takes all the hearty, familiar flavors and combines them into a healthy meal. Using sprouted beans helps lower the alkalinity. Make a double batch and freeze the left-overs—if you have any! Be sure to use diced tomatoes and pasta sauce that contain no sugar, meat, or dairy.

Recipe Tip Fresh cilantro and dried cilantro have vastly different flavors. If you don't have fresh on hand, omit it altogether from the recipe.

Cooking spray
1 small onion, chopped
1 cup diced red bell pepper
2 garlic cloves, finely chopped
2 cups sprouted beans (see page 201),
  black, kidney, or pinto
1 (14.5-ounce) can diced tomatoes

2 tablespoons Homemade Barbecue Sauce
  (page 207)
1 (8-ounce) jar organic pasta sauce
¼ cup organic salsa, mild, medium, or hot
¼ cup organic fresh cilantro
Dash chili powder
Dash ground cumin

1. Spray a medium-size pot with cooking spray. Set it over medium heat. Add the onions and sauté for 5 minutes, or until they're soft and slightly caramelized.
2. Add the bell pepper, garlic, sprouted beans, tomatoes, Homemade Barbecue Sauce, pasta sauce, salsa, cilantro, chili powder, and cumin. Stir to combine. Simmer for 20 minutes.
3. Serve immediately.

Serves 4. Prep time: 5 minutes. Cook time: 25 minutes

PER SERVING (1 CUP): CALORIES: 101 / TOTAL FAT: 2.7G / CARBOHYDRATES: 18.5G / FIBER: 5.3G / PROTEIN: 3.9G

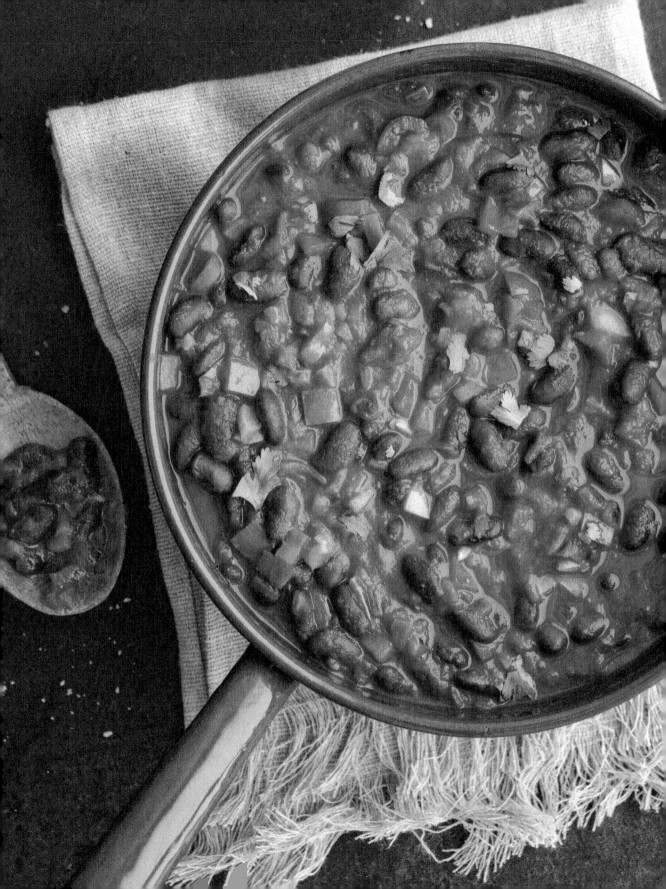

STIR-FRY VEGETABLES

QUICK
& EASY

IMMUNITY
BOOST

THYROID
SUPPORT

KIDNEY
SUPPORT

This is about as easy as it gets. The secret to success is your *mise en place*—literally, everything in place. So chop all the vegetables and measure all the ingredients to organize yourself before you start cooking. Also, use a large enough pan so the vegetables aren't crowded; otherwise they'll be soggy.

2 tablespoons coconut oil

1 red bell pepper, cored, seeded, and julienned

1 yellow bell pepper, cored, seeded, and julienned

½ cup thinly sliced red onion

1 cup sliced yellow squash

1 cup small broccoli florets

2 cups sliced bok choy

1 cup fresh mung bean sprouts

½ cup snow peas

1 garlic clove, minced

¼ teaspoon sea salt

½ cup Asian Citrus Dressing (page 209)

2 tablespoons sesame oil

1. In a wok or large skillet set over medium-high heat, add the coconut oil and heat for 1 to 2 minutes.
2. While stirring constantly, add the red bell pepper, yellow bell pepper, and onion.
3. Add the yellow squash, broccoli, bok choy, bean sprouts, and snow peas. Stir-fry for 2 minutes. Stir in the garlic and salt.
4. Add the dressing and stir to combine.
5. Remove from the heat and stir in the sesame oil.
6. Serve immediately.

Serves 2. Prep time: 5 minutes. Cook time: 5 minutes

PER SERVING (2 CUPS): CALORIES: 354 / TOTAL FAT: 12.8G / CARBOHYDRATES: 24.1G / FIBER: 8.4G / PROTEIN: 8.4G

VEGETABLE POTPIE

IMMUNITY
BOOST

THYROID
SUPPORT

KIDNEY
SUPPORT

These individually baked potpies are going to surprise you. They have the same hearty flavor you expect from a chicken potpie, but with none of the acid-producing dairy or animal products in them. If you don't have individual ramekins, just use a regular casserole dish, but cook it a little longer. You can tell it's done when the crust is a light golden brown and starts to crack slightly.

Cooking spray

1 large sweet potato, peeled and chopped into ½-inch pieces

1 large carrot, peeled and finely chopped

1 celery stalk, finely chopped

1 medium onion, finely chopped

1 large shiitake mushroom, or 4 to 5 white mushrooms, chopped

¾ cup chopped broccoli florets (optional)

⅓ cup frozen peas

4 to 6 garlic cloves, finely chopped

2 cups vegetable broth

1 to 2 teaspoons sea salt

1 teaspoon dried oregano

1 bay leaf

Pinch red pepper flakes

1 All-Purpose Pie Crust (page 181)

1. Preheat the oven to 350°F.
2. Spray a medium skillet with cooking spray. Place the pan over medium heat and add the sweet potato, carrot, celery, onion, mushrooms, broccoli, peas, and garlic. Sauté the vegetables for 5 minutes, or until slightly softened.
3. Add the broth, salt, oregano, bay leaf, and red pepper flakes. Simmer the mixture for about 5 minutes, or until thickened and bubbly. Remove from the heat and cool slightly.
4. Divide the vegetable mixture evenly among four individual ramekins.
5. Roll the pie dough to a ¼-inch thickness. Cut the dough into circles slightly larger than the ramekins.
6. Top each ramekin with one dough disc. Press the edges down to seal. With a sharp knife, cut an opening in the top to let steam escape while cooking.

continued →

Vegetable Potpie *continued*

7. Place the filled ramekins on a baking sheet and into the preheated oven. Bake for 15 minutes. Remove from the oven and cool slightly.
8. Serve warm.

Serves 4. Prep time: 15 minutes. Cook time: 25 minutes

PER SERVING (1 INDIVIDUAL POTPIE): CALORIES: 195 / TOTAL FAT: 4.1G / CARBOHYDRATE: 247.1G / FIBER: 4.5G / PROTEIN: 7.1G

DATE NIGHT GARLIC BAKE

IMMUNITY
BOOST

THYROID
SUPPORT

KIDNEY
SUPPORT

This recipe is called Date Night Garlic Bake because both of you have to eat it! Otherwise, if only one person eats this much garlic, the other might deem you unkissable. Garlic has so many health benefits, including lowered cholesterol and decreased cancer risk. But, mostly, it's just delicious.

1 pound broccoli, cut into bite-size pieces

4 carrots, peeled and sliced

3 garlic heads, cloves peeled and chopped, or 3 tablespoons minced

2 teaspoons lemon zest

1 teaspoon sea salt

¼ teaspoon mustard powder

1 cup vegetable broth

2 tablespoons coconut oil

1. Preheat the oven to 400°F.
2. In a medium bowl, stir together the broccoli, carrots, garlic, lemon zest, salt, mustard powder, broth, and coconut oil.
3. Evenly spread the mixture into a baking pan. Cover with aluminum foil and place in the preheated oven. Bake for 30 minutes, stirring once.
4. Serve immediately.

Serves 2. Prep time: 10 minutes. Cook time: 30 minutes

PER SERVING (2 CUPS): CALORIES: 270 / TOTAL FAT: 15.2G / CARBOHYDRATES: 28.1G / FIBER: 5.1G / PROTEIN: 11.6G

LAYERED RATATOUILLE

IMMUNITY
BOOST

KIDNEY
SUPPORT

Classic ratatouille is a French casserole-style dish with rich eggplant and savory herbs. This version modernizes the French classic using less fat. And the layered vegetables make a stunning presentation. Bring this one out for company and they'll think you're channeling Julia Child!

Cooking spray

½ onion, chopped

2 garlic cloves, minced

1 (6-ounce) can tomato paste

4 tablespoons coconut oil, divided

¾ cup water

½ teaspoon sea salt

1 small eggplant, thinly sliced

1 zucchini, thinly sliced

1 yellow squash, thinly sliced

1 red bell pepper, thinly sliced

1 yellow bell pepper, thinly sliced

2 large tomatoes, thinly sliced

1 teaspoon fresh thyme leaves

1. Preheat the oven to 375°F.
2. Spray a small skillet with cooking spray. Set the pan over medium heat, add the onion and garlic, and sauté for 5 minutes, or until soft. Remove from the heat and set aside.
3. In a small bowl, combine the tomato paste, onion mixture, 1 tablespoon coconut oil, and the water. Season with the salt. Spread this mixture along the bottom of a baking dish.
4. In a large bowl, add the eggplant, zucchini, yellow squash, red bell pepper, yellow bell pepper, tomatoes, tomatoes, and 1 tablespoon coconut oil. Toss to evenly coat all the vegetables.
5. Following the inside edge of the baking dish and working inward, top the tomato mixture with the vegetables, in layers and alternating by types (e.g., 1 slice of eggplant, then 1 zucchini slice, 1 squash slice, 1 red bell pepper slice, 1 yellow pepper slice, and finally, 1 tomato slice). Repeat the spiral layers until all vegetables are used.

6. Season with the thyme and finish by drizzling the remaining 2 tablespoons coconut oil over the vegetables. Cover with aluminum foil, or parchment paper, and place in the preheated oven.

7. Bake for about 30 minutes, or until the vegetables are tender and fully roasted.

Serves 4. Prep time: 15 minutes. Cook time: 35 minutes

PER SERVING (¼ FINISHED RECIPE): CALORIES: 208 / TOTAL FAT: 14.4G / CARBOHYDRATES: 19.1G / FIBER: 7.9G / PROTEIN: 3.6G

IMMUNITY
BOOST

THYROID
SUPPORT

KIDNEY
SUPPORT

THANKSGIVING ANYTIME ROASTED VEGETABLES

This dish will make your entire kitchen smell as if it were Thanksgiving—even in July! The combination of winter squashes, carrots, and apples is a classic fall combination. The key to success in this recipe is to cut all the vegetables about the same size. Fresh sage can be found in the refrigerator section of the market, and it is a critical ingredient to make it taste like the holidays.

1 butternut squash, peeled and cubed

1 baking pumpkin, peeled and cubed

2 large carrots, peeled and cubed

2 green apples, peeled, cored, and sliced

3 fresh sage leaves, finely chopped

1 teaspoon sea salt

2 teaspoons coconut oil

1. Preheat the oven to 350°F.
2. In a large bowl, combine the butternut squash, pumpkin, carrots, apples, sage, salt, and coconut oil. Toss to coat evenly in the oil and seasonings. Transfer the vegetables to a roasting pan, in a single layer.
3. Roast for 60 minutes, stirring occasionally. Serve.

Serves 4. Prep time: 15 minutes. Cook time: 60 minutes

PER SERVING (1 CUP): CALORIES: 176 / TOTAL FAT: 12.4G / CARBOHYDRATES: 44.3G / FIBER: 6.3G / PROTEIN: 4.1G

NO BS BRUSSELS SPROUTS

QUICK
& EASY

IMMUNITY
BOOST

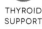

THYROID
SUPPORT

KIDNEY
SUPPORT

This Thai-inspired dish is the real deal. Healthy Brussels sprouts are quickly roasted and tossed with a coconut-ginger sauce. You might just love this sauce so much you start putting it on everything. Even vegetables you don't think you like!

For the sauce
½ cup light unsweetened coconut milk
1 teaspoon freshly squeezed lime juice
1½ teaspoons ground ginger
½ teaspoon chili-garlic sauce
1 packet stevia

For the Brussels sprouts
¾ pound Brussels sprouts, ends removed, trimmed, and halved
1 tablespoon coconut oil
½ teaspoon sea salt

To make the sauce:

In a medium saucepan set over medium heat, combine the coconut milk, lime juice, ground ginger, chili-garlic sauce, and stevia. Bring ingredients to a simmer. Cook for 5 minutes. Remove from the heat and set aside.

To make the Brussels sprouts:

1. Preheat the broiler.
2. In a medium bowl, add the Brussels sprouts, coconut oil, and sea salt. Toss to combine.
3. Transfer to a medium cast-iron pan or ovenproof skillet. Sauté over medium heat for 5 minutes.
4. Place the skillet under the broiler and broil for 3 minutes, or until the leaves are slightly browned.
5. Transfer the Brussels sprouts to a medium bowl. Add the sauce and toss to coat. Serve immediately.

Serves 2. Prep time: 5 minutes. Cook time: 10 minutes

PER SERVING (6 OUNCES BRUSSELS SPROUTS WITH ¼ CUP SAUCE): CALORIES: 169 / TOTAL FAT: 8.7G / CARBOHYDRATES: 19.4G / FIBER: 6.5G / PROTEIN: 7.9G

QUICK
& EASY

IMMUNITY
BOOST

KIDNEY
SUPPORT

GRILLED VEGETABLE STACK

You won't believe how easy these gorgeous sandwiches are. The portobello mushrooms form a base to hold the creamy hummus. The rest of the vegetables are grilled to a roasty, caramelized perfection and layered on top. When eating the rainbow, this is your pot of gold at the end.

2 portobello mushrooms, stemmed and
  gills removed
½ eggplant, sliced into ¼-inch-thick slices
1 yellow bell pepper, seeded and sliced
  lengthwise

1 red bell pepper, seeded and sliced
  lengthwise
1 red onion, peeled and sliced
½ cup Healthy Hummus (page 103), divided
1 teaspoon sea salt, divided

1. Preheat the grill or a broiler.
2. Over medium coals or a gas flame (or under a broiler, if using), grill the mushroom caps, eggplant, yellow bell peppers, red bell peppers, and onion for 20 minutes, turning occasionally.
3. Fill one mushroom cap with ¼ cup of hummus. Top with half of the eggplant, half of the yellow peppers, half of the red peppers, and half of the onion slices. Sprinkle ½ teaspoon of salt on top. Set aside.
4. Repeat with the second mushroom cap and remaining ingredients. Serve warm.

Serves 2. Prep time: 10 minutes. Cook time: 20 minutes

PER SERVING (1 VEGETABLE STACK WITH ¼ CUP HUMMUS): CALORIES: 179 / TOTAL FAT: 3.1G / CARBOHYDRATES: 15.7G / FIBER: 3.6G / PROTEIN: 3.9G

BBB SOUP

QUICK
& EASY

IMMUNITY
BOOST

THYROID
SUPPORT

KIDNEY
SUPPORT

This soup contains three hearty ingredients that will fill you up: bok choy, a leafy Asian vegetable; broccolini, a relative of broccoli; and brown rice. It's an ideal combination of nutrition and flavor and it comes together in minutes.

3 cups vegetable broth

1 cup chopped bok choy

1 bunch broccolini, chopped roughly

½ cup cooked brown rice

In a medium saucepan set over medium heat, place the broth, bok choy, broccolini, and brown rice. Bring to a simmer and cook for 10 minutes, or until the vegetables are cooked until tender. Serve.

Serves 2. Prep time: 5 minutes. Cook time: 10 minutes

PER SERVING (2 CUPS): CALORIES: 172 / TOTAL FAT: 3.5G / CARBOHYDRATES: 38.5G / FIBER: 2.7G / PROTEIN: 11.7G

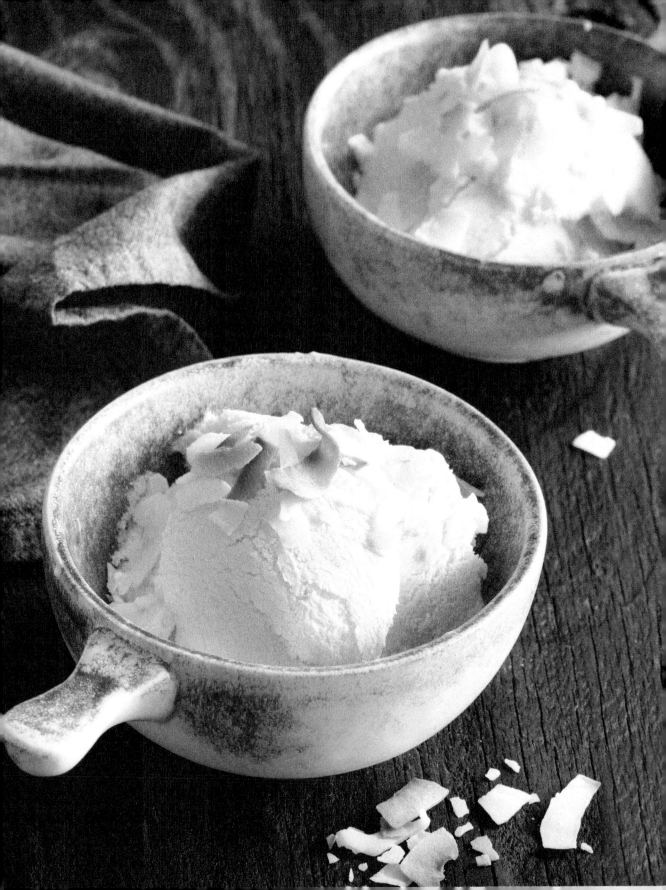

10

DELIGHTFUL DESSERTS

ALL-PURPOSE PIE CRUST

QUICK
& EASY

IMMUNITY
BOOST

THYROID
SUPPORT

KIDNEY
SUPPORT

This pie crust is a basic recipe that's good for either sweet or savory pies. If you're making a savory pie, leave the recipe as is. If you're making a sweet pie, add ½ cup coconut sugar. It's a good idea to pre-bake your pie crust when making a recipe that requires baking, or it will get soggy.

Recipe Tip You can chill the dough before rolling out so it's easier to work with.

1 cup almond flour

1 tablespoon coconut oil

⅛ teaspoon sea salt

1. Line an 8-inch pie pan with parchment paper.
2. In a food processor, combine the almond flour, coconut oil, and salt. Mix until a ball forms.
3. Place the dough ball in the middle of the parchment-lined pie plate. Top with a second sheet of parchment paper.
4. With your hands, press the crust evenly over the bottom and up the sides of the pan. Remove the top piece of parchment paper, but leave the one under the crust.
5. Pre-bake, if needed.

To pre-bake your crust, after lining your pie pan with the crust, place the pan into a baking pan filled with about 1-inch of water (a water bath). This will keep the pan from direct contact with the heat and the almond flour from burning. Carefully transfer the water-filled baking pan to a preheated 350°F oven and bake for 10 minutes.

Serves 8. Prep time: 15 minutes

PER SERVING (⅛ OF PIE CRUST): CALORIES: 84 / TOTAL FAT: 7.6G / CARBOHYDRATES: 2.5G / FIBER: 1.4G / PROTEIN: 2.5G

QUICK
& EASY

IMMUNITY
BOOST

THYROID
SUPPORT

KIDNEY
SUPPORT

COCONUT ICE CREAM SUNDAE

This is going to become one of your go-to recipes. Coconut milk forms an ice cream that is then topped with your favorite toppings. If you don't have time to freeze this overnight, freeze some canned, full-fat coconut milk in ice cube trays. Then, just drop them in your blender and you'll be eating ice cream in no time.

Recipe Tip This recipe calls for a lot of sugar. If you prefer your dessert to be less sweet, you can adjust the amount. And, instead of freezing overnight, you can make this in your ice cream maker and process according to your machine's instructions.

2 (13-ounce) cans full-fat unsweetened coconut milk

1 cup coconut sugar

⅛ teaspoon sea salt

1 vanilla bean, split lengthwise and seeds scraped out

Toppings of choice (bananas, shredded unsweetened coconut, chopped almonds, strawberries)

1. In a blender, blend together the coconut milk, coconut sugar, salt, and vanilla bean seeds. Transfer the mixture to a freezer-safe bowl. Freeze overnight.
2. Place two scoops of the ice cream in a small bowl. Garnish with your favorite alkaline-friendly toppings. Serve.

Note The coconut ice cream does not freeze solid, but is scoopable.

Serves 4. Prep time: 5 minutes. Freezing time: overnight (or use an ice cream maker)

PER SERVING (1 CUP ICE CREAM WITHOUT TOPPINGS): CALORIES: 306 / TOTAL FAT: 22.7G / CARBOHYDRATES: 30.8G / FIBER: 2.6G / PROTEIN: 2.2G

WARM PEACH COBBLER

QUICK
& EASY

IMMUNITY
BOOST

THYROID
SUPPORT

KIDNEY
SUPPORT

This cobbler is technically a crisp. But, topped with Coconut Ice Cream (page 182), your mouth will be too full to say cobbler or crisp. Don't use canned peaches here, as they are too mushy. Use fresh, frozen, or thawed peaches.

Recipe Tip To peel peaches quickly, dunk each one in boiling water (using tongs) for about 30 seconds. The skin should peel right off.

Cooking spray

2 pounds peaches, peeled and
  roughly chopped

1 packet stevia

1 vanilla bean, split lengthwise and seeds
  scraped out

¼ teaspoon cinnamon

1½ cups raw almonds

½ cup shredded unsweetened coconut

1 tablespoon coconut oil, melted

¼ teaspoon sea salt

1. Preheat the oven to 350°F.
2. Spray a 9-inch baking dish with cooking spray.
3. In a large saucepan over medium heat, combine the peaches, stevia, vanilla bean, and cinnamon. Stir well until the mixture comes to a boil. Remove from the heat.
4. In a food processor, combine the almonds, coconut, coconut oil, and salt. Pulse until a sticky, crumbly mixture forms.
5. Transfer the peaches to the prepared baking dish. Top with the almond-coconut mixture.
6. Bake in the preheated oven for 15 minutes, or until the top is lightly golden. Serve warm.

Serves 6. Prep time: 15 minutes. Cook time: 15 minutes

PER SERVING (1 CUP): CALORIES: 240 / TOTAL FAT: 16.8G / CARBOHYDRATES: 20.8G / FIBER: 5.8G / PROTEIN: 6.6G

THANKSGIVING PUDDING

IMMUNITY
BOOST

THYROID
SUPPORT

KIDNEY
SUPPORT

This recipe is basically a crustless pumpkin pie with other fruits added. If you want a real pie, use the All-Purpose Pie Crust (page 181) with this recipe. Frankly, this nutrition-packed pudding is great on its own.

Recipe Tip You can make your own pumpkin purée very easily by baking small "baking pumpkins" (not the Halloween carving kind). It's a good idea to scoop out the seeds first. You can roast those for the Party Mix (page 100)!

1 (15-ounce) can unsweetened
  pumpkin purée
½ cup unsweetened coconut milk
1 teaspoon cinnamon
½ teaspoon nutmeg

¼ teaspoon sea salt
½ cup raisins
½ cup apples, peeled, cored, and diced
Coconut Whipped Cream (page 202), for
  serving (optional)

1. Preheat the oven to 350°F.
2. In a food processor, blend the pumpkin, coconut milk, cinnamon, nutmeg, and salt until aerated.
3. Add the raisins and apples. Pulse just to combine. Pour the mixture into a 9-inch baking dish.
4. Bake in the preheated oven for 60 minutes, or until the top cracks slightly.
5. Serve warm with a dollop of Coconut Whipped Cream (if using).

Serves 8. Prep time: 10 minutes. Baking time: 60 minutes

PER SERVING (¾ CUP): CALORIES: 69 / TOTAL FAT: 0.6G / CARBOHYDRATES: 16.1G / FIBER: 2.2G / PROTEIN: 1.4G

DON'T SLIP BANANA SPLITS

QUICK
& EASY

IMMUNITY
BOOST

THYROID
SUPPORT

KIDNEY
SUPPORT

Can you even believe there's a recipe for banana splits in this cookbook? And this recipe is so healthy it won't make you slip from your diet. Feel free to top it with any toppings of your choice, as long as they're on the Go list.

Recipe Tip Other ideas for toppings include fruit preserves, almond butter, and fresh strawberries.

1 large banana, peeled and halved
  lengthwise
2 scoops Coconut Ice Cream (page 182)
2 tablespoons toasted, shredded,
  unsweetened coconut

1 tablespoon toasted, chopped almonds
¼ cup Coconut Whipped Cream (page 202)
1 dark cherry, stem on

1. In a single-serving dish, place the banana. Add the ice cream between the banana halves.
2. Top with the coconut, almonds, and whipped cream.
3. Crown with the cherry on top and serve.

Serves 1. Prep time: 10 minutes

PER SERVING: CALORIES: 393 / TOTAL FAT: 21.6G / CARBOHYDRATES: 47.6G / FIBER: 6.6G / PROTEIN: 6.6G

VALENTINE'S DAY DATES

QUICK
& EASY

IMMUNITY
BOOST

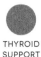

THYROID
SUPPORT

KIDNEY
SUPPORT

One of the hardest things for many people to give up on this diet is chocolate. This recipe uses dates so naturally sweet you'll get your sugar rush without the guilt. Note that the recipe serves one—this is for the lonely hearts on Valentine's Day. You can double it if you've got a real date to eat dates.

Recipe Tip If you can't find pitted dates, they are very easy to pit yourself. Just use a sharp knife to slice the date lengthwise. Remove the pit and proceed with the recipe.

4 pitted Medjool dates

4 almond halves, divided

¼ cup shredded unsweetened coconut

1. With a sharp knife, slice the dates lengthwise without cutting all the way through, so the halves are still connected.
2. Press open the dates and lay them on a flat surface. Use a rolling pin to flatten each date. Place one almond half on one side of a flattened date. Fold the other side over to enclose the almond between the date halves. Repeat with remaining dates and almonds.
3. Press each date into the coconut.
4. Eat and enjoy!

Serves 1. Prep time: 10 minutes

PER SERVING (4 DATES): CALORIES: 178 / TOTAL FAT: 8G / CARBOHYDRATES: 27.5G / FIBER: 4.3G / PROTEIN: 2G

MELON MADNESS

QUICK
& EASY

IMMUNITY
BOOST

THYROID
SUPPORT

KIDNEY
SUPPORT

Watermelon is one of the most alkalizing foods in the world. This recipe combines watermelon with other delicious melons to create an easy, elegant dessert. If you don't feel like showing off, skip the "melon bowl" and simply serve this in a regular serving bowl. Or, get creative with your watermelon bowl and carve it like a basket!

Recipe Tip Summertime is a great time to experiment with different fruits. Have fun and add some exotic melons to this dish.

½ lengthwise-cut watermelon, flesh scooped into balls, shell reserved

1 cup bite-size honeydew melon pieces
1 cup bite-size cantaloupe pieces

In a large bowl, combine the watermelon balls, honeydew, and cantaloupe. Transfer the fruit to the watermelon shell and serve.

Use a melon baller to make the watermelon balls in a jiffy.

Serves 4. Prep time: 15 minutes

PER SERVING (½ CUP): CALORIES: 31 / TOTAL FAT: 0.2G / CARBOHYDRATES: 7.4G / FIBER: 0.7G / PROTEIN: 0.8G

SUMMER FRUIT CRISP

QUICK
& EASY

IMMUNITY
BOOST

THYROID
SUPPORT

KIDNEY
SUPPORT

This dish is very similar to the Warm Peach Cobbler (page 183). Unlike that recipe, this dish lets you use whatever fruits are fresh from the harvest. A quick trip to the farmers market will show what's at the peak freshness of the season. Just be sure you stick to foods on the Go list.

Recipe Tip Top your Don't Slip Banana Split (page 185) or Coconut Ice Cream Sundae (page 182) with this fruit for an even more decadent dessert.

Cooking spray

2 cups chopped summer fruits, like strawberries and plums

1 packet stevia

1 vanilla bean, split lengthwise and seeds scraped out

1½ cups raw almonds

½ cup shredded unsweetened coconut

1 tablespoon coconut oil, melted

¼ teaspoon sea salt

1. Preheat the oven to 350°F.
2. Spray a 9-inch baking dish with cooking spray.
3. In a large saucepan over medium heat, combine the chopped fruits, stevia, and vanilla bean seeds. Stir until the mixture comes to a boil. Remove from the heat.
4. In a food processor, combine the almonds, coconut, coconut oil, and salt. Pulse until a sticky, crumbly mixture forms.
5. Transfer the fruits to the prepared baking dish. Top with the almond-coconut mixture.
6. Bake in the preheated oven for 15 minutes, or until the top is lightly golden.
7. Serve warm.

Serves 6. Prep time: 15 minutes. Cook time: 15 minutes

PER SERVING (½ CUP): CALORIES: 240 / TOTAL FAT: 16.8G / CARBOHYDRATES: 20.8G / FIBER: 5.8G / PROTEIN: 6.6G

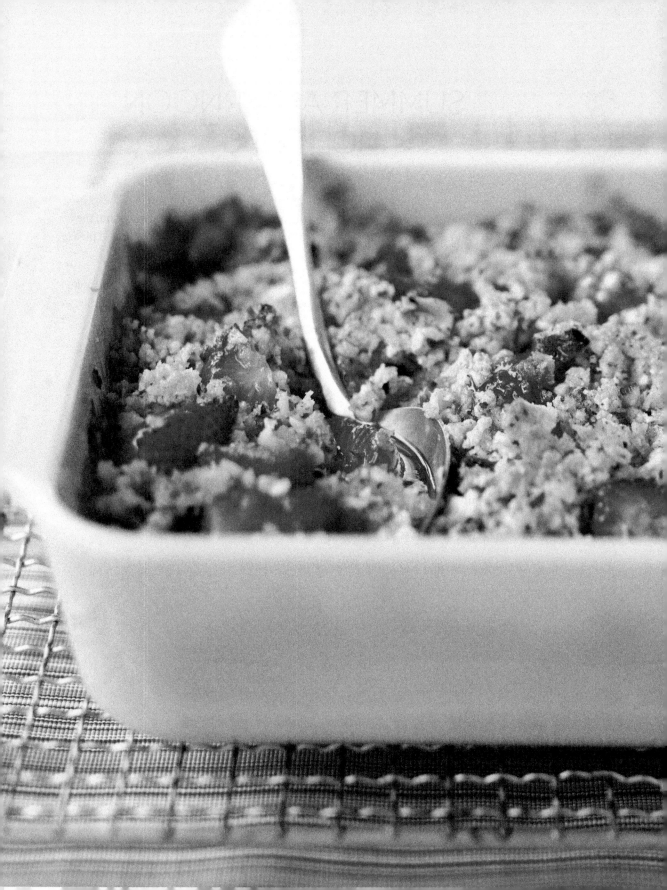

QUICK
& EASY

IMMUNITY
BOOST

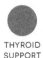

THYROID
SUPPORT

KIDNEY
SUPPORT

SUMMER AFTERNOON ICE POPS

These ice pops are easier to make than chasing down the ice cream truck. And, they are dairy- and sugar-free, too. Use any fresh fruits you like. This cool treat will please adults and kids alike.

Recipe Tip If you don't have ice pop molds, get some! Until then, though, you make these in ice cube trays and cover with plastic wrap. Stick toothpicks in the middle before freezing.

1 (13-ounce) can unsweetened coconut milk

1 packet stevia

1 vanilla bean, split lengthwise and seeds scraped out

1½ cups chopped fresh fruit

1. In a small bowl, mix together the coconut milk, stevia, and vanilla bean seeds.
2. Evenly divide the chopped fruit among the ice pop molds. They will be partially filled.
3. Pour the coconut milk mixture over the fruit, gently shaking each mold to settle the milk.
4. Insert the ice pop handles into the molds. Freeze until completely frozen, about 2 hours.

Serves 6. Prep time: 5 minutes. Freezing time: 2 hours

PER SERVING (1 ICE POP): CALORIES: 163 / TOTAL FAT: 14.1G / CARBOHYDRATE: 7.1G / FIBER: 4.2G / PROTEIN: 2.5G

NO-BAKE FIG NEWTONS

QUICK
& EASY

IMMUNITY
BOOST

THYROID
SUPPORT

KIDNEY
SUPPORT

These cookies don't look a thing like their packaged counterparts. But they are so beautiful they could easily be included in a gift tin of holiday cookies. They're nutritious, too. Just be careful not to eat the whole batch at once!

Recipe Tip For a more elegant presentation, flatten each cookie ball and press an almond half into the center of each.

3 cups dried figs, stemmed

1 cup raw almonds

1 vanilla bean, split lengthwise and seeds scraped out

½ teaspoon sea salt

1. In a food processor, combine the figs, almonds, vanilla bean seeds, and salt. Pulse until a dough forms.
2. Scoop the dough by tablespoonfuls and roll into balls by hand.
3. Refrigerate in an airtight container for up to one week.

Serves 12. Prep time: 15 minutes

PER SERVING (1 COOKIE): CALORIES: 170 / TOTAL FAT: 4.4G / CARBOHYDRATES: 32.3G / FIBER: 5.1G / PROTEIN: 3.6G

CRISPY RICE TREATS

QUICK
& EASY

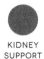

IMMUNITY
BOOST

THYROID
SUPPORT

KIDNEY
SUPPORT

These rice treats are definitely on your 20 percent list because of the rice. But compared to the original, these are still delicious and healthy. Make them once in a while when you want to feel like a kid again—or share them with your actual kids!

Recipe Tip These treats don't contain marshmallow because marshmallow contains gelatin, an animal byproduct. You can find brown rice syrup in your local health food store.

Cooking spray

⅔ cup brown rice syrup

¼ cup coconut oil

1 vanilla bean, split lengthwise and seeds
  scraped out

¼ teaspoon sea salt

4 cups brown rice crisp cereal

1. Spray a 9-inch baking pan with cooking spray.
2. In a medium saucepan set over medium heat, combine the brown rice syrup and coconut oil. Bring to a boil and boil for 1 minute. Stir in the vanilla bean seeds and salt.
3. In a large bowl, add the rice cereal. Pour the syrup mixture over the cereal. Mix with a wooden spoon to combine thoroughly.
4. Transfer the rice mixture to the prepared pan. Spray your hands with cooking spray and use them to press gently on the rice mixture to distribute it evenly in the pan.
5. Refrigerate for 45 minutes.
6. When ready to eat, bring to room temperature, cut into 12 bars, and serve.

Serves 12. Prep time: 5 minutes. Cook time: 1 minute. Chilling time: 45 minutes

PER SERVING (1 BAR): CALORIES: 104 / TOTAL FAT: 4.6G / CARBOHYDRATES: 15.8G / FIBER: 4.6G / PROTEIN: 0.3G

DATE-SPICE PUDDING

QUICK
& EASY

IMMUNITY
BOOST

THYROID
SUPPORT

KIDNEY
SUPPORT

This pudding is as easy to make as 1, 2, 3. It tastes like the holidays, but without the extra fat and calories that come from figgy pudding. Depending on the size of your blender, you may need to make this in two batches. It will keep in the refrigerator for a few days.

Recipe Tip If you're not familiar with whole nutmeg, it comes in glass jars and looks like nuts, and is commonly available in any grocery store's spice section.

1¾ cups almond milk

1½ teaspoons apple cider vinegar

1¼ cups pitted Medjool dates, quartered

½ cup coconut oil

1½ teaspoons cinnamon

1½ teaspoons ginger

¼ teaspoon freshly grated whole nutmeg

1 vanilla bean, split lengthwise and seeds
   scraped out

1 teaspoon sea salt

1. In a medium bowl, combine the almond milk and cider vinegar. Let sit for 10 minutes until the milk curdles.
2. In a blender, add the dates, coconut oil, cinnamon, ginger, nutmeg, vanilla bean seeds, and sea salt. Top with the milk mixture. Process until smooth.
3. Pour the pudding into an airtight container and chill, or serve immediately.

Don't worry about the curdled milk. It hasn't gone bad. This serves to thicken the pudding.

Serves 1. Prep time: 15 minutes

PER SERVING: CALORIES: 304 / TOTAL FAT: 19.8G / CARBOHYDRATES: 32.8G /
FIBER: 3.8G / PROTEIN: 3.3G

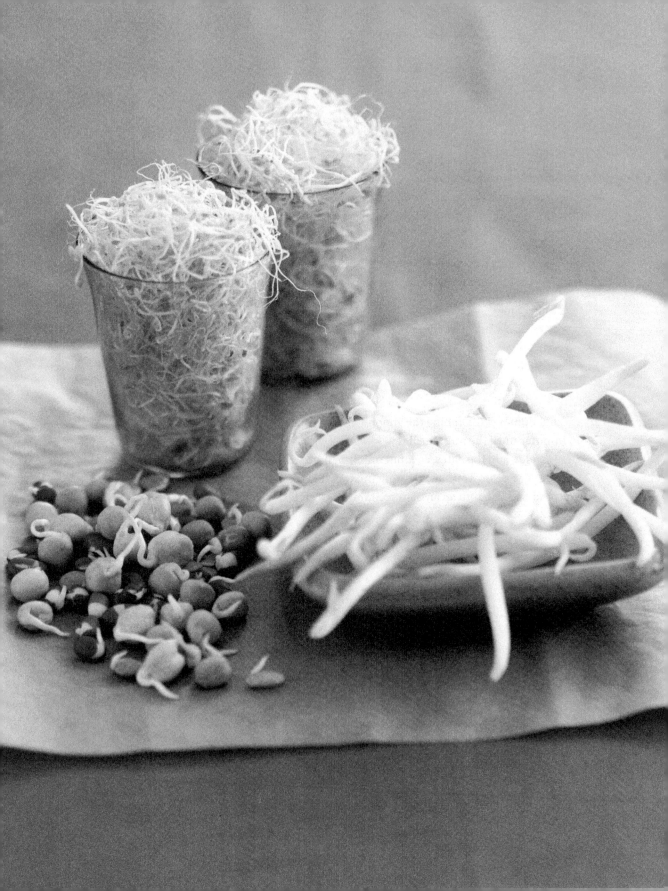

11

KITCHEN STAPLES

CONDIMENTS, SAUCES, AND DRESSINGS

HOMEMADE KETCHUP

QUICK
& EASY

IMMUNITY
BOOST

KIDNEY
SUPPORT

You might be wondering why on earth you'd want to make your own ketchup. After all, it's easy enough to buy. The reason is that store-bought or restaurant ketchup usually contains high-fructose corn syrup, one of the most acid-producing ingredients on the planet. This recipe is just as good as the other kinds, without all the nastiness.

Recipe Tip If you freeze this, you might want to run it through a blender after defrosting to remix all the ingredients to the desired consistency, as it will separate.

1 (6-ounce) can unsweetened tomato paste

½ cup brown rice syrup

½ cup apple cider vinegar

1 packet stevia

¼ teaspoon onion powder

⅛ teaspoon garlic powder

1. In a saucepan set over medium heat, combine the tomato paste, brown rice syrup, cider vinegar, stevia, onion powder, and garlic powder. Whisk until smooth.
2. Bring the mixture to a boil. Lower the heat and simmer for 25 minutes, stirring frequently.
3. Chill and serve cold.

Serves 12. Prep time: 5 minutes. Cook time: 25 minutes

PER SERVING (1 TABLESPOON): CALORIES: 51 / TOTAL FAT: 0.1G / CARBOHYDRATES: 13.4G / FIBER: 0.7G / PROTEIN: 1G

SALSA FRESCA

QUICK
& EASY

IMMUNITY
BOOST

KIDNEY
SUPPORT

This is a great way to use up those end-of-summer tomatoes. Since the recipe is uncooked, use the sweetest onions you can find. Also, the cumin seed is important—try to use that instead of ground. This salsa is even better the next day!

Recipe Tip Play with spices by adding a seeded, chopped jalapeño or chipotle pepper. Just remember to wear gloves so you don't accidentally get spices in your nose or eyes.

4 fully ripened tomatoes, diced

½ sweet onion (Maui or Vidalia), diced

1 tablespoon toasted cumin seeds

¼ cup chopped fresh cilantro

¼ cup apple cider vinegar

½ teaspoon sea salt

In a large airtight container, mix together the tomatoes, onion, cumin seeds, cilantro, cider vinegar, and salt. Cover and chill for 15 minutes so the flavors blend before serving.

Serves 6. Prep time: 20 minutes

PER SERVING (¼ CUP): CALORIES: 25 / TOTAL FAT: 0.4G / CARBOHYDRATE: 4.6G / FIBER: 1.2G / PROTEIN: 1.5G

HAWAIIAN SALSA

QUICK
& EASY

IMMUNITY
BOOST

KIDNEY
SUPPORT

This is another recipe that's a variation on a theme. In this one, we start with the basic Salsa Fresca (page 198) and add pineapple and mango to it. This gives it an island flavor that goes great with any of the coconut recipes in the book. Just a reminder that the tomatoes are not allowed if you're following the Thyroid-Support Plan, so consider that when pairing this with other recipes.

Recipe Tip You can use canned, fresh, or frozen pineapple in this recipe. If all you have on hand is frozen pineapple, just be sure to thaw it before using.

4 fully ripened tomatoes, diced

½ sweet onion (Maui or Vidalia), diced

½ cup diced fresh mango

½ cup diced pineapple

¼ cup apple cider vinegar

½ teaspoon sea salt

In a large airtight container, mix together the tomatoes, onion, mango, pineapple, cider vinegar, and salt. Cover and chill for 15 minutes so the flavors blend before serving.

Serves 6. Prep time: 20 minutes

PER SERVING (¼ CUP): CALORIES: 48 / TOTAL FAT: 0.2G / CARBOHYDRATES: 5.3G / FIBER: 1.4G / PROTEIN: 0.9G

GREAT GRAVY

QUICK
& EASY

IMMUNITY
BOOST

THYROID
SUPPORT

KIDNEY
SUPPORT

Everyone loves a good gravy, but most are made with dairy, wheat, and animal-based broth. This version has none of those things, and all of the taste! Practice with this recipe a bit before serving it to company. Even "regular" gravy takes some practice.

Recipe Tip If you do burn the flour, throw it out and start over. There's no rescuing it. Live and learn!

1 tablespoon coconut oil, melted
2 tablespoons coconut flour
½ cup vegetable broth

2 tablespoons almond milk
½ teaspoon sea salt

1. In a saucepan set over medium heat, gently heat the coconut oil. Don't let it get too hot or the flour will instantly burn.
2. Add the coconut flour and whisk to make a thick paste.
3. Slowly whisk in the vegetable broth. Bring to a boil and let it boil for 4 minutes, or until thickened.
4. Reduce the heat to low. Add the almond milk and salt. Continue cooking until the desired consistency.
5. Serve warm.

Serves 6. Prep time: 5 minutes. Cook time: 10 minutes

PER SERVING (¼ CUP): CALORIES: 35 / TOTAL FAT: 2.5G / CARBOHYDRATES: 2.8G / FIBER: 0.8G / PROTEIN: 1.8G

SPROUTED BEANS

QUICK
& EASY

IMMUNITY
BOOST

THYROID
SUPPORT

KIDNEY
SUPPORT

Sprouting beans is a way to reduce their acidic effects, and, it's easy to do. You probably made these in grade school. Only make enough so they'll be eaten in a couple of days.

Recipe Tip If you don't feel like going to all this trouble, you can buy sprouted beans at most health food stores. But, hey, try it yourself at least once!

1 cup dried beans of choice
½ teaspoon sea salt

1. Rinse and soak the beans overnight in enough water to cover and the sea salt.
2. In the morning, drain the beans and rinse them in a colander set over a bowl or in the sink. Cover the beans.
3. Rinse and drain the beans several times a day until the beans begin to sprout. This should take 3 to 4 days, depending on the type of bean.
4. Store in the refrigerator for a day or two.

Serves 4. Prep time: 3 to 4 days, depending on the type of bean

PER SERVING (¼ FINISHED RECIPE): CALORIES: 10 / CARBOHYDRATES: 2G /
FIBER: 0.9G / PROTEIN: 0.5G

COCONUT WHIPPED CREAM

QUICK
& EASY

IMMUNITY
BOOST

THYROID
SUPPORT

KIDNEY
SUPPORT

This recipe is going to be the one that made you glad you bought this book. Seriously—whipped cream that isn't made from dairy? The key to success here is to refrigerate the can of coconut milk overnight, upside down, so the cream is at the top of the can when you open it. Only use the solidified part of the coconut cream, not the water.

Recipe Tip Coconut milk takes longer to whip than whipping cream. Just be patient! Also, if you want to make it sweeter, use coconut sugar instead of stevia.

1 (13-ounce) can full-fat unsweetened coconut milk, chilled

1 packet stevia

1 vanilla bean, split lengthwise and seeds scraped out

1. Open the can of coconut milk. Use a spoon to scoop out the thick layer of coconut milk fat. Place it into a large bowl. Using a whisk or hand mixer, beat just as you would regular whipping cream, until fluffy.
2. Add the stevia and vanilla bean seeds and whip for another minute or so.
3. Use immediately or store covered in the refrigerator for one to two days.

Serves 8. Prep time: 15 minutes

PER SERVING (¼ CUP): CALORIES: 197 / TOTAL FAT: 21.2G / CARBOHYDRATES: 2.8G / FIBER: 0.1G / PROTEIN: 2G

APPLE BUTTER

IMMUNITY
BOOST

THYROID
SUPPORT

KIDNEY
SUPPORT

This is fantastic spread on any of the muffins in this cookbook. It takes a while to make, but your whole house will smell like fall. And it's packed with fiber and nutrients.

Recipe Tip You can use apple cider in place of apple juice for this recipe, but choose some with no added sugar. Also, do not use the cinnamon or spices in this recipe if you do.

4 pounds apples, peeled, cored, and chopped

2 cups fresh apple juice

1 tablespoon freshly squeezed lemon juice

2 packets stevia

1 teaspoon cinnamon

1 vanilla bean, split lengthwise and seeds scraped out

Pinch ground cloves

1. In a large pot, combine the apples, apple juice, and lemon juice. Bring to a simmer and cook for 1 hour, until soft. Remove from the heat and cool slightly.
2. Using an immersion blender (or your regular blender in batches), purée the apples until smooth.
3. Add the stevia, cinnamon, vanilla bean seeds, and cloves to the apples. Return the pot to the heat and cook for an additional 2 hours, stirring frequently.
4. Cool the apple butter. Transfer to an airtight container and refrigerate.

Serves 24. Prep time: 10 minutes. Cook time: 3 hours

PER SERVING (2 TABLESPOONS): CALORIES: 49 / TOTAL FAT: 0.2G / CARBOHYDRATES: 12.9G / FIBER: 1.9G / PROTEIN: 0.2G

SUN-DRIED TOMATO SAUCE

QUICK
& EASY

IMMUNITY
BOOST

KIDNEY
SUPPORT

This uncooked sauce can be put on a salad, or warmed and used with any of the Italian recipes in this book. Be sure to use sun-dried tomatoes not packed in oil. The oil adds a ton of calories and it's not on the Go list. If the sun-dried tomatoes are hard, soak them in a little water before using.

Recipe Tip The tomato paste is the key to the intense tomato flavor here. Don't leave it out.

1 cup cherry tomatoes, halved

½ cup tightly packed sun-dried tomatoes

3 tablespoons coconut oil

⅓ cup fresh basil

1 tablespoon tomato paste

1 teaspoon sea salt

1 teaspoon garlic powder

1. In a food processor, combine the cherry tomatoes, sun-dried tomatoes, coconut oil, basil, tomato paste, salt, and garlic powder.
2. Pulse to combine until the desired consistency is reached.

Serves 4. Prep time: 10 minutes

PER SERVING (½ CUP): CALORIES: 132 / TOTAL FAT: 12.2G / CARBOHYDRATES: 6.1G / FIBER: 1.5G / PROTEIN: 1.4G

ENCHILADA SAUCE

QUICK
& EASY

IMMUNITY
BOOST

KIDNEY
SUPPORT

This sauce is so delicious you're going to want to dip everything in it. Once you taste this, you'll never buy the canned stuff again. Freeze some so you have it on hand.

Recipe Tip Add a tablespoon of Dutch-processed cocoa powder before cooking to add a depth of flavor reminiscent of a mole sauce.

2 tablespoons coconut oil

2 tablespoons coconut flour

2 tablespoons chili powder

2 cups water

1 (8-ounce) can tomato paste

1 teaspoon garlic powder

½ teaspoon cumin

½ teaspoon onion powder

½ teaspoon sea salt

¼ teaspoon red pepper flakes

1. In a medium pot set over medium heat, heat the coconut oil, coconut flour, and chili powder. Cook for 1 minute so the flour doesn't taste raw.
2. Add the water, tomato paste, garlic powder, cumin, onion powder, salt, and red pepper flakes, to taste. Bring the mixture to a simmer and cook for 25 minutes, stirring occasionally.
3. Serve warm.

Serves 8. Prep time: 5 minutes. Cook time: 26 minutes

PER SERVING (½ CUP): CALORIES: 68 / TOTAL FAT: 3.6G / CARBOHYDRATES: 8.3G / FIBER: 1.6G / PROTEIN: 1.8G

WHITE SAUCE

QUICK
& EASY

IMMUNITY
BOOST

THYROID
SUPPORT

KIDNEY
SUPPORT

This is another staple sauce that can go over just about anything. It's great on vegetables and on top of bowls. As with the gravy, practice a little so you can get it just right. Then, amaze your friends with this healthy sauce.

Recipe Tip Once you've mastered the sauce base, you can add all kinds of seasonings to it to change it up. Try adding basil or fresh rosemary, or use it to make a mushroom soup. The options are almost endless.

1 tablespoon coconut oil

3 tablespoons coconut flour

2¼ cups almond milk

1 teaspoon sea salt

1 teaspoon garlic powder

1 teaspoon onion powder

1. In a saucepan set over medium heat, gently heat the coconut oil. Don't let it get too hot or the flour will instantly burn.
2. Add the coconut flour and whisk to make a thick paste.
3. Add the almond milk and bring to a boil. Boil for 2 minutes, then lower heat.
4. Add the salt, garlic powder, and onion powder. Simmer until thickened.
5. Serve warm.

Serves 6. Prep time: 5 minutes. Cook time: 10 minutes

PER SERVING (½ CUP): CALORIES: 83 / TOTAL FAT: 4.1G / CARBOHYDRATES: 8.1G / FIBER: 0.5G / PROTEIN: 3.5G

HOMEMADE BARBECUE SAUCE

QUICK & EASY

IMMUNITY BOOST

KIDNEY SUPPORT

What is summertime without a good barbeque? This sauce tastes fantastic on grilled veggies, but doesn't contain the acid-producing sugar that bottled sauces have. Feel free to play around with this recipe, adding fruit or spices to it. It will keep in the refrigerator for about a week.

Recipe Tip This is particularly good when made with peaches or mango. Just add ¼ cup when cooking for a sweet, fruity flavor.

2 cups water

1 onion, chopped

1 (8-ounce) can tomato sauce

¼ cup apple cider vinegar

2 teaspoons paprika

2 teaspoons chili powder

1 packet stevia

1. In a medium saucepan, combine the water, onion, tomato sauce, cider vinegar, paprika, chili powder, and stevia. Bring the ingredients to a full boil.
2. Reduce the heat and simmer for 20 minutes.
3. Serve immediately, or cool and refrigerate in an airtight container.

Serves 6. Prep time: 5 minutes. Cook time: 25 minutes

PER SERVING (2 TABLESPOONS): CALORIES: 36 / TOTAL FAT: 0.8G / CARBOHYDRATES: 7G / FIBER: 2.3G / PROTEIN: 1.3G

CILANTRO SALAD DRESSING

QUICK
& EASY

IMMUNITY
BOOST

THYROID
SUPPORT

KIDNEY
SUPPORT

Each of the salad dressing recipes in this chapter is an easy variation on a theme—one part apple cider vinegar to two parts coconut oil, with different seasonings. The good news is that you'll quickly get the hang of making your own salad dressing and won't feel the need to buy the expensive, salty, acid-producing ones in the store. Have fun and play around with these recipes.

Recipe Tip Don't use dried cilantro or coriander in this recipe. It doesn't taste remotely the same. Pick the freshest cilantro you can find and rinse it well. Cut off the stems if you prefer.

½ cup coconut oil

¼ cup apple cider vinegar

½ cup chopped fresh cilantro

1 teaspoon freshly squeezed lemon juice

¼ teaspoon sea salt

½ packet stevia

In a blender, add the coconut oil, cider vinegar, cilantro, lemon juice, salt, and stevia. Blend until the cilantro is fully incorporated and the oil and vinegar emulsify.

Serves 12. Prep time: 5 minutes

PER SERVING (2 TABLESPOONS): CALORIES: 80 / TOTAL FAT: 9.1G / CARBOHYDRATES: 0.1G / FIBER: 0.4G / PROTEIN: 0.3G

ASIAN CITRUS DRESSING

QUICK
& EASY

IMMUNITY
BOOST

THYROID
SUPPORT

KIDNEY
SUPPORT

This dressing can be used with any of the Asian dishes in this cookbook. It's also great over a bowl of quinoa and steamed vegetables. You want to use ground ginger and garlic powder in this recipe instead of fresh. Otherwise, the taste is too sharp.

Recipe Tip If you prefer the sharp taste of fresh ginger and garlic then, by all means, use fresh. Just grate them into the blender.

½ cup coconut oil

¼ cup apple cider vinegar

1 tablespoon freshly squeezed orange juice

1 tablespoon dark sesame oil

3 tablespoons chopped scallions

2 teaspoons toasted sesame seeds

½ teaspoon ground ginger

½ teaspoon garlic powder

¼ teaspoon sea salt

½ packet stevia

1. In a blender, combine the coconut oil, cider vinegar, orange juice, sesame oil, scallions, sesame seeds, ginger, garlic powder, sea salt, and stevia.
2. Blend until the ingredients are well mixed and the oil and vinegar emulsify.

Serves 12. Prep time: 5 minutes

PER SERVING (2 TABLESPOONS): CALORIES: 90 / TOTAL FAT: 1.1G / CARBOHYDRATES: 1.1G / FIBER: 1.4G / PROTEIN: 0.9G

AVOCADO SALAD DRESSING

QUICK
& EASY

IMMUNITY
BOOST

THYROID
SUPPORT

KIDNEY
SUPPORT

This is a great recipe to make if you've got avocados that need to be used. Choose ones that are on the soft side for best flavor. This goes very well with the Mexican recipes in this book. It's got a ton of flavor, so you won't need much to pack a flavorful punch.

Recipe Tip If you like it spicy, add a jalapeño while blending.

½ cup coconut oil

¼ cup apple cider vinegar

1 avocado, peeled and pitted

¼ cup chopped fresh cilantro

1 teaspoon freshly squeezed lime juice

1 teaspoon garlic powder

1 teaspoon cumin

1 teaspoon onion powder

¼ teaspoon sea salt

½ packet stevia

In a blender, combine the coconut oil, cider vinegar, avocado, cilantro, lime juice, garlic powder, cumin, onion powder, sea salt, and stevia. Blend until all ingredients are mixed well and the oil and vinegar emulsify.

Serves 12. Prep time: 5 minutes

PER SERVING (2 TABLESPOONS): CALORIES: 101 / TOTAL FAT: 10.8G / CARBOHYDRATES: 1.2G / FIBER: 0.9G / PROTEIN: 0.2G

RANCH DRESSING

QUICK
& EASY

IMMUNITY
BOOST

THYROID
SUPPORT

KIDNEY
SUPPORT

The key to this recipe is the raw cashews that have been soaked in water for 2 hours and drained. Cashews, when prepared this way, make for a very creamy tasting base. This recipe should be on your 20 percent list, since cashews are less alkalizing than almonds. Serve cold for the best results.

Recipe Tip If you want to make a chipotle-ranch dressing, add one-half of a chipotle pepper while blending, or to taste.

1 cup raw cashews, soaked for 2 hours
  and drained

¼ cup freshly squeezed lemon juice

¼ cup apple cider vinegar

2 tablespoons diced red onion

1 tablespoon finely chopped scallions

1 teaspoon garlic powder

½ teaspoon sea salt

½ packet stevia

1 tablespoon chopped fresh parsley

½ teaspoon finely chopped fresh dill

1. In a blender, combine the cashews, lemon juice, cider vinegar, red onion, scallions, garlic powder, salt, and stevia. Purée until smooth and creamy.
2. Add the parsley and dill. Pulse quickly just to combine.
3. Refrigerate in an airtight container. Chill for 1 hour before serving.

Serves 12. Prep time: 2 hours, 10 minutes. Chilling time: 1 hour

PER SERVING (2 TABLESPOONS): CALORIES: 70 / TOTAL FAT: 5.3G / CARBOHYDRATES: 4.3G / FIBER: 3.3G / PROTEIN: 1.9G

ALKALINE–ACID FOOD CHART

EXTREMELY ALKALINE

Baking soda
Lemons
Lentils
Limes
Lotus root
Mineral water

Nectarines
Onions
Persimmons
Pineapple
Sea salt
Sea vegetables

Seaweed
Seeds, pumpkin
Sweet potato
Tangerines
Taro root
Watermelon

MODERATELY ALKALINE

Alfalfa sprouts
Apple, sweet
Avocados
Banana, ripe
Beets
Bell pepper
Broccoli
Cabbage
Cayenne
Cantaloupe
Carob
Cauliflower
Celery
Currants
Dates
Figs, fresh
Fruit juices
Garlic

Ginger, fresh
Grapefruit
Grapes, less sweet
Grapes, sour
Grapes, sweet, seeded
  and seedless
Green beans, fresh
Guavas
Kiwifruit
Lettuce, leafy green
Lettuce, pale green
Mangoes
Melons
Oranges
Papayas
Parsley
Passion fruit
Peaches, less sweet

Peaches, sweet
Pear, less sweet
Pear, sweet
Pears, fresh, sweet
Pears, less sweet
Potato, with skin
Pumpkin, less sweet
Pumpkin, sweet
Raisins
Raspberries
Squash
Strawberries
Sweet corn, fresh
Turnip
Vegetable juices
Vinegar, apple cider
Umeboshi plums
Watercress

SLIGHTLY ALKALINE

Almonds
Apple, sour
Apricots
Artichoke,
  Jerusalem
Arugula
Asparagus
Avocado oil
Blackberries
Brussels sprouts
Carrots
Cashews
Cherries
Chestnuts
Chestnuts,
  dry roasted
Chive
Cilantro
Citrus
Coconut, fresh
Coconut oil
Collard greens
Cucumbers

Dewberry
Eggplant
Endive
Ginseng
Herbs, most
Honey, raw
Honeydew melon
Japonica rice
Kale
Kabocha
Kohlrabi
Leeks
Loganberries
Mushrooms
Mustard greens
Oats
Oil, flax
Oil, olive
Okra
Olives
Parsnips
Pickles,
  homemade

Quinoa
Radishes
Rice syrup
Rutabaga
Seeds, most
Sesame seeds
Spices
Sprouts
Tea, ginger
Tea, green
Tea, mu
Tomatoes,
  less sweet
Tomatoes, sweet
Turnip greens
Unsulfured molasses
Vinegar, sweet brown rice
Vinegar, umeboshi
Whole sprouted grains
Wild rice
Yeast, nutritional

SLIGHTLY ACIDIC

Amaranth
Beans, fava
Beans, string
Beans, wax
Black-eyed peas
Chutney
Curry
Dried fruit

Guava
Honey
Kasha
Maple syrup
Oil, canola
Oil, grape seed
Oil, pumpkin seed
Oil, sunflower

Pine nuts
Rice, brown
Rhubarb
Spinach
Vinegar
Zucchini

Alcohol
Bananas, green
Barley groats
Beans, aduki
Beans, lima
Beans, navy
Beans, pinto
Beans, red
Beans, white
Blueberries
Bran
Buckwheat
Butter
Casein
Cereals, unrefined
Chard
Cheese, cottage
Cheese, soy
Cheeses, aged
Chicken
Chickpeas
Coconut, dry
Corn
Crackers, unrefined rice
Crackers, unrefined rye
Crackers, unrefined wheat
Cranberries
Dried beans, adzuki
Dried beans, kidney
Dried beans, mung
Dried beans, pinto
Egg whites
Eggs, whole, hard cooked
Farina

Fructose
Game
Goose
Green peas
Honey, pasteurized
Kamut
Ketchup
Lard
Legumes, other
Maize
Maple syrup,
  unprocessed
Milk, cow's
Milk, goat's, raw
Milk, goat's,
  homogenized
Milk, homogenized
Milk, soy
Milk protein
Molasses, unsulfured
  and organic
Mussels
Mustard
Mutton
Nutmeg
Nuts, most
Oat bran
Oil, almond
Oil, chestnut
Oil, palm kernel
Oil, safflower
Oil, sesame
Olives, pickled
Pasta, whole grain

Pastry, whole grain
  and honey
Peanuts
Pecan
Pistachio
Plums
Pomegranates
Popcorn, with salt
  and/or butter
Potato
Prunes
Rice, basmati
Rice, white
Rye
Seeds, pumpkin
Seeds, sunflower
Seitan
Semolina
Shellfish
Snow peas
Soy sauce
Spelt
Squid
Tapioca
Teff
Tofu
Tomatoes
Turkey
Vanilla
Veal
Vinegar, balsamic
Wheat
Wheat bread,
  sprouted organic

EXTREMELY ACIDIC

Artificial tabletop
   sweeteners, like
   NutraSweet, Spoonful,
   Sweet 'N Low, Equal,
   or Aspartame
Barley
Beef
Beer
Brazil nuts
Bread
Brown sugar
Carbonated soft
   drinks, especially
   the cola type
Cereals, refined
Cheese, processed
Chocolate
Cigarettes and
   tobacco
Cocoa
Coffee

Cream of wheat,
   unrefined
Custard, with
   white sugar
Fish
Flour, white, wheat
Fried foods
Fruit juices with sugar
Hazelnuts
Ice cream
Jams, jellies
Lamb
Liquor
Lobster
Malt
Maple syrup,
   processed
Molasses, sulfured
Oil, cottonseed
Pasta, white

Pastries and cakes
   from white flour
Pheasant
Pickles, commercial
Pork
Poultry
Pudding
Seafood
Soybeans
Sugar, white
Table salt, refined
   and iodized
Tea, black
Venison
Vinegar, white, processed
Walnuts
White bread
Whole-wheat foods
Wine
Yeast
Yogurt, sweetened

DIRTY DOZEN AND CLEAN 15

If you are committed to eating healthy food, then heaps of fruits and vegetables are a huge part of your meals. One of the questions that will crop up is whether to buy organic or not. Most commercially grown produce is contaminated to a certain degree with chemicals and pesticides that can have damaging effects on your health. So organic food is a logical choice if you have an eye on longevity and wellness.

Unfortunately, organic fruits and vegetables can be expensive and unavailable in some areas. This means you have to pick and choose which organic produce to buy. A nonprofit environmental watchdog organization called Environmental Working Group (EWG) makes this choice a little easier. The EWG looks at data supplied by the U.S. Department of Agriculture and the U.S. Food and Drug Administration regarding pesticide residues and compiles a list each year outlining the pesticide loads found in commercial crops. You can use these lists to decide which fruits or vegetables to buy organic (the "Dirty Dozen") in order to minimize your exposure to pesticides and which produce is considered safe enough to purchase conventionally grown (the "Clean 15"). These lists change every year, so make sure to look up the most recent before you fill your shopping cart.

THE DIRTY DOZEN

APPLES

CELERY

CHERRY TOMATOES

CUCUMBERS

GRAPES

NECTARINES (IMPORTED)

PEACHES

POTATOES

SNAP PEAS (IMPORTED)

SPINACH

STRAWBERRIES

SWEET BELL PEPPERS

Plus produce contaminated with highly toxic organophosphate insecticides:

BLUEBERRIES (DOMESTIC)

HOT PEPPERS

There is also a list from the EWG that outlines foods that have the least pesticide contamination and can be purchased from commercially grown crops. This does not mean they are pesticide-free, so wash these fruits and vegetables thoroughly.

THE CLEAN 15

ASPARAGUS

AVOCADOS

CABBAGE

CANTALOUPE (DOMESTIC)

CAULIFLOWER

EGGPLANT

GRAPEFRUIT

KIWI

MANGOS

ONIONS

PAPAYAS

PINEAPPLES

SWEET CORN

SWEET PEAS (FROZEN)

SWEET POTATOES

It is important to remember that the positive impact of eating a diet rich in fruits and vegetables far outweighs the risk of pesticide exposure.

MEASUREMENT CONVERSIONS

Volume Equivalents (Liquid)

U.S. Standard	U.S. Standard (ounces)	Metric (approximate)
2 tablespoons	1 fl. oz.	30 mL
¼ cup	2 fl. oz.	60 mL
½ cup	4 fl. oz.	120 mL
1 cup	8 fl. oz.	240 mL
1½ cups	12 fl. oz.	355 mL
2 cups or 1 pint	16 fl. oz.	475 mL
4 cups or 1 quart	32 fl. oz.	1 L
1 gallon	128 fl. oz.	4 L

Volume Equivalents (Dry)

U.S. Standard	Metric (approximate)
⅛ teaspoon	0.5 mL
¼ teaspoon	1 mL
½ teaspoon	2 mL
¾ teaspoon	4 mL
1 teaspoon	5 mL
1 tablespoon	15 mL
¼ cup	59 mL
⅓ cup	79 mL
½ cup	118 mL
⅔ cup	156 mL
¾ cup	177 mL
1 cup	235 mL
2 cups or 1 pint	475 mL
3 cups	700 mL
4 cups or 1 quart	1 L
½ gallon	2 L
1 gallon	4 L

Oven Temperatures

Fahrenheit (F)	Celsius (C) (approximate)
250	120
300	150
325	165
350	180
375	190
400	200
425	220
450	230

Weight Equivalents

U.S. Standard	Metric (approximate)
½ ounce	15 g
1 ounce	30 g
2 ounces	60 g
4 ounces	115 g
8 ounces	225 g
12 ounces	340 g
16 ounces or 1 pound	455 g

REFERENCES

Abbas, Abul K., Andrew H. Lichtman, and Shiv Pillai. *Basic Immunology: Functions and Disorders of the Immune System*. 4th ed. Philadelphia: Saunders, 2012.

American Autoimmune Related Diseases Association, Inc. "Autoimmune Statistics." Accessed June 15, 2014. http://www.aarda.org /autoimmune-information/autoimmune -statistics/.

Koufman, Jamie A., and Nikki Johnston. "Potential Benefits of pH 8.8 Alkaline Drinking Water as an Adjunct in the Treatment of Reflux Disease." *Annals of Otology, Rhinology & Laryngology* 121, no.7 (July 2012): 431–4. http://evamor.com /static/pdf/koufman_1242.pdf.

National Institute of Diabetes and Digestive and Kidney Diseases. "Diet for Kidney Stone Prevention." NIH Publication. 6425, no.13 (February 2013). http://kidney.niddk.nih.gov/kudiseases /pubs/kidneystonediet/Kidney_Stone_Diet _508.pdf.

Schwalfenberg, G. K. "The Alkaline Diet: Is There Evidence That an Alkaline pH Diet Benefits Health?" *Journal of Environmental and Public Health* 2012 (2012): 727630. doi:10.1155/2012/727630.

RESOURCES

ALMOND MEAL/FLOUR
www.bobsredmill.com

COCONUT FLOUR
www. bobsredmill.com

COCONUT OIL
http://nutiva.com

COCONUT SUGAR
http://madhavasweeteners.com

COCONUT TORTILLAS AND WRAPS
http://thepurewraps.com

DUTCH-PROCESSED COCOA POWDER
www.drugstore.com

SEA VEGETABLES
http://kelpnoodles.com

SUPERFOODS
http://ultimatesuperfoods.com

GLOSSARY

80/20 rule: Part of the acid-alkaline balance that says that 80 percent of one's food should be alkalizing and 20 percent can be acidifying.

acid: A substance with a pH of less than 7.

acid-alkaline balance: The dietary ratio of acidifying foods to alkalizing foods.

acidifying: Foods that, regardless of their pH level, test as acidic after the ash test is performed.

alkaline: A substance with a pH of greater than 7.

alkalizing: Foods that, regardless of their pH level, test as alkaline after the ash test is performed.

ash test: A test to determine the alkalizing or acidifying effect of a substance. It's performed by burning the substance and then mixing the ash residue with water and measuring the pH of the liquid.

Dutch-processed cocoa: Cocoa processed in such a way as to make it more alkaline.

eating the rainbow: A term that means to eat fresh foods that are of every color in the spectrum.

immune-support diet: A diet that enhances the body's immune system. It's a diet rich in vitamins and minerals.

immune system: The body's defense against bacteria, viruses, and other invaders. Through a series of steps called the immune response, the immune system attacks organisms and substances that invade body systems and cause disease.

kidney: One of a pair of organs in the body that processes and excretes urine.

kidney stone: A stone-like formation in the kidneys that can interfere with the passage of urine out of the body.

kidney-support diet: A diet that causes urine to be more alkaline and less likely to form kidney stones.

nightshade vegetables: The plant family Solanaceae, including belladonna, eggplant, nightshade, peppers of the genus *Capsicum*, petunia, potato, tobacco, and tomato. The chemical makeup of these foods has the potential to cause inflammation in the body. They are to be avoided if on a thyroid-supporting diet.

neutral: A substance with a pH of 7.

pH: An acronym for "potential hydrogen." It refers to the degree of concentration of hydrogen ions in a substance or solution. It is designated on a scale from 0 to 14. Higher numbers mean a substance is more alkaline in nature and has a greater potential for absorbing more hydrogen ions.

thyroid: The gland in the neck that secretes hormones that regulate metabolism.

thyroid-support diet: A diet that supports the thyroid's functioning by avoiding foods in the nightshade family.

INDEX

CPSIA information can be obtained at www.ICGtesting.com
Printed in the USA
BVOW10s1536060116

431988BV00005B/12/P